Crashing the Boards

A Friendly Study Guide for the USMLE Step 1

Crashing the Boards

A Friendly Study Guide for the USMLE Step 1

2nd edition

Benjamin Yeh

Sean Wu

Matt Flynn

Shankha S. Biswas

Ketan R. Bulsara

Lawrence Liao

Joseph A. Paydarfar

LIPPINCOTT WILLIAMS & WILKINS
A **Wolters Kluwer** Company

Editor: Elizabeth Nieginski
Managing Editor: Marette D. Magargle-Smith
Marketing Manager: Jennifer Conrad

351 West Camden Street
Baltimore, Maryland 21201-2436 USA

227 East Washington Square
Philadelphia, PA 19106

Printed in the United States of America

First Edition, 1996
Second Edition, 1999

The publishers have made every effort to trace the copyright holders for borrowed material. If they have inadvertently overlooked any, they will be pleased to make the necessary arrangements at the first opportunity.

To purchase additional copies of this book, call our customer service department at **(800) 638-3030** or fax orders to **(301) 824-7390**. International customers should call **(301) 714-2324**.

99 00 01 02 03
1 2 3 4 5 6 7 8 9 10

Dedication

————————————— *To our families, friends,*
and the Duke University
Medical School Class of 1996.

And to everyone facing
the USMLE Step 1 exam.

Preface

Dear fellow students,

In these pages we assemble the notes and mnemonics that students found most useful in studying for the most recent USMLE Step 1 exams. We cover the highest of the high yield, including several obscure but heavily tested facts. This book is designed to earn you many quick points on the Boards. It is also designed to guide studying and to enhance the value of other study materials. It is not a comprehensive review of the basic sciences.

Our goal in writing this book is to present material in the most direct, concise, and memorable way possible. To this end, we employ the following organization principles:

- Information is presented using a variety of mnemonics, diagrams, and tables.
- Information is broken down into discrete, easily digestible "nuggets."
- Important points are spelled out in diagrams so that you do not have to skip back and forth between text and picture.
- For each major subject area we provide Coach's Tips to illustrate the emphasis of the USMLE Step 1 exam.
- Key words and concepts are boldfaced for rapid review.

Crashing the Boards was made possible by the collaborative efforts of numerous students who recently took the USMLE Step 1 exam. This book was originally assembled by an intramural basketball team at Duke University Medical School. A guiding principle then and now is that teamwork can overcome daunting obstacles and can bring much benefit to many. If you find this book useful and would like to contribute to it or be a chapter author of the next edition, please contact us at the address below. Please note that if you would like to be a chapter author, try to contact us before you take the USMLE.

Crashing the Boards
c/o Ben Yeh
24 Jefferson Ave.
Tenafly, NJ 07670
email:
benyeh@itsa.ucsf.edu

We wish you the best of luck on the USMLE Step 1 exam.

Sincerely,

The Authors

Acknowledgments

We are indebted to the contributions of numerous colleagues, friends, and family. In particular, we wish to acknowledge Maryam Hendi Paydarfar for her computer graphics and design expertise, her emotional support, and her fine cooking.

To Joseph Corless, MD, PhD, we owe a huge debt for his model basic science instruction. Dr. Corless' humor, encouragement, coffee, and advice on education and teaching greatly enhanced the quality of this book. We also thank Samuel E. George, MD, and Dale Purves, MD, for the generous use of their computer facilities, without which the first editions of this book would not have been possible.

To Lynn Anthony, Christopher Gammard, and Theresa Flynn, we owe many thanks. Their work and contributions to the first edition of this book are greatly appreciated.

We owe many thanks to Mark Routbort, Harvey Cohen, MD, and the Duke University Medical School chapter of Alpha Omega Alpha for generous funding of the pilot editions of *Crashing the Boards*. In addition, we wish to thank the Duke University Medical School classes of 1997, 1998, and 1999 for their ideas and support for this book.

Thanks also to the many students from across the United States who contributed to the candid student-to-student review book evaluations found in the appendix. These data should prove useful for the next generation of test-takers.

Several students wrote in to offer ideas for this current edition of *Crashing the Boards*. Many thanks for helping to make this guide more useful for test-takers. In particular, we thank Bella L. Orbino for her close reading of the text and suggestions and Jay B. Rao for his assistance on the Microbiology and Immunology chapter revisions.

Contents

Cover design by Maryam Hendi Paydarfar

Strategy

CHAPTER 1

Introduction

One of the first rites of passage every new practicing physician must face is the USMLE Step 1. Although it is not as life-changing as, say, getting married for the first time, it can be just as stressful.

The USMLE covers an enormous amount of material. A typical biochemistry book is about two inches thick and weighs about as much as a small human head. On top of that, there are six additional subjects to cover. That's a lot of information to put into a three pound human brain.

Although mastery of every topic covered by the USMLE Step 1 exam is virtually impossible, one can perform very well by learning a smaller well-selected set of information. *Crashing the Boards* was written by medical students who had just taken the USMLE Step 1. Our goal is to maximize your test score.

This book is a concise high-yield study guide in three parts. The introduction of the book and the Coach's Tips in each chapter reveal student-to-student advice designed to streamline your studies and gear them toward exam-relevant material. The body of each subject chapter is a compilation of the highest yield facts that will help make sure you get the easy points. The appendix is a frank student-to-student guide to other review books available for the USMLE Step 1 based on surveys of students who actually used these books.

What Does the USMLE Step 1 Really Test?

The USMLE Step 1 covers the basic sciences fundamental to modern medicine. The subject areas include anatomy (including embryology and histology), biochemistry, human behavior (including epidemiology), microbiology, pathology, pharmacology, and physiology. The most heavily emphasized topics have been biochemistry, microbiology, and pharmacology, closely followed by physiology and pathology.

The USMLE Step 1 emphasizes basic science that is relevant to clinical medicine and pathology. For example, questions regarding the coagulation cascade will likely focus on the reactions and factors involved in bleeding disorders or steps that can be affected by drugs. The test will not ask about the fascinating crystal structure of these factors or their melting points.

The USMLE Step 1 also stresses *areas of overlap* between subjects. For example, the biochemistry of glucose metabolism will certainly be tested because it overlaps with the pathology of diabetes and the pharmacology of oral hypoglycemics. Likewise, drugs that have known effects on physiology will almost certainly be tested, often repeatedly.

Basic Information on the Exam

The United States Medical Licensing Examinations are required for Board certification. To be licensed to practice medicine in the United States, a physician must pass all three steps. The first two steps are traditionally taken prior to beginning internship. The third step is usually taken during residency. With few exceptions, "Board certification" in a field requires passing all three USMLE exams, completing an accredited residency, and passing field-specific exams. Eventually, foreign medical graduates will also have to pass a Clinical Skills Assessment given solely in English and using standardized patients.

Early registration is required. A passport photo, application form, and check payable in U.S. dollars on a U.S. bank must be received roughly three months before the exam.

The USMLE Step 1 Exam takes two days. There are two three-hour sessions a day, with one test booklet per session. An examinee must break the seals on all four test booklets for his or her exam to be scored. Each booklet contains a table of normal lab values. Please note that future USMLE exams after 1999 are expected to be administered through a computer interface, and the format may change accordingly.

In recent exams, each booklet has contained 151 to 181 questions. The test employs three types of questions. The first 120 to 150 questions use the one-best-answer format. Each question has four or five options. The next few questions use the EXCEPT format. Test instructions will make it clear when the EXCEPT questions begin. The final section gives lists of 4 to 26 answers with one or more associated questions. These matching questions typically ask you to identify a structure labeled on a diagram or to choose the best drug from a list.

The last booklet, given during the afternoon session of the second day, contains several color photographs. The photographs typically show gross pathology specimens and color slides. Corresponding questions often give clinical information and ask for a diagnosis.

Coach's Tips—Preparing for the Boards

Just how much time you will need to study for the USMLE Step 1 exam depends on you. How much do you know? How fast can you cram? How efficiently do you study? And most importantly, how well do you want to do? Talk to people who have taken the exam to get a feel for the test. Do not believe people who say the exam is easy.

Probably the most critical point is to **study what you do not know.** Do not spend a lot of time studying the finer points of your best subject areas. If you are good at biochemistry, study other subjects first. Or at least, study those high-yield topics in biochemistry that are less familiar to you. If you took your basic science courses long ago, we suggest paying special attention to pharmacology and immunology. These subject areas have changed the most.

Using review books and notes

Be selective with the books and notes you use. Review books are valuable in large part because they are concise. Choose books short enough that you can learn the material in the time you have. At the same time, don't underestimate your ability to learn. If you used a good review book as the text for a basic science course, then by all means read it again.

Note that although review books are excellent summaries, sometimes they give only cursory coverage of key topics. For this reason, try to keep a standard text open and available for quick reference in order to double cover these points.

Set up a schedule

Schedules allow you be more realistic with your studying. A weekly calendar will let you pace your studying and reveal how much or little time you can afford to master each topic.

Try to decide when to study each subject. Some subjects, particularly microbiology and pharmacology, are more easily forgotten and should be reviewed closer to the exam. It also helps immensely to save several days at the end for reviewing high-yield material such as your notes and this book.

The daily study routine

Set realistic daily studying goals. During the weeks before the Boards, studying may well be foremost on your mind. However, very few people can study effectively all day for weeks on end. Leave time for working out, socializing, and whatever else you like to do. If you *actually study hard* for four or six hours, you can learn a large amount of material in a day.

As you plan out your days, try to put your best brain forward. If you are a morning person, then study in the morning. If you tend to get sluggish after lunch, use that time to run errands or socialize. Many people find that they study best late at night. Others feel more satisfied if they get all of their studying done early and then take every evening off.

Effective study strategies make a big difference. A few boldfaced words are in order. Memory can be enhanced by **active learning, integration, variety,** and **self-testing.**

- **Active learning.** Avoid the common pitfall of mindlessly running your highlighter over material. Rather, glance through the chapters to get an overview. Read selected portions closely and **reorganize the information** as needed for your own use. Take **brief** notes, draw diagrams, or make charts to force yourself to process and integrate information. The mnemonics or diagrams that **you make up** are the easiest to remember.
- **Integration.** As you study a topic, think about how it relates to others. For example, as you study cardiovascular drugs, refer often to cardiovascular and renal physiology. By doing this you will learn more efficiently and will reinforce information that you have already learned. You will also get a higher score, because topics that overlap between subjects are emphasized on the Boards.
- **Variety.** Do whatever it takes to keep your mind engaged. Supplement your study with flashcards, study in groups, study in different places, or use self-tests and class notes in addition to review books. Tailor your note-taking technique to the material at hand. Microbiology facts, for example, often fit well into tables or tree diagrams, whereas flow diagrams often work best for biochemistry.

- **Self-testing.** As you study, take time to review in your mind the material just covered. Try to re-draw diagrams from memory and recall what you have learned. The combination of integration and self-testing is highly effective. Practice questions and tests can be very useful, particularly for identifying areas of weakness. Keep in mind, however, that practice tests and retired test questions don't always reflect USMLE Step 1 exam content, formats, or difficulty.

How to Use *Crashing the Boards*

- Before you start studying, we recommend reading this introduction as well as the Coach's Tips found at the beginning of each chapter. This will help you determine your study strategy as you tackle other study materials.
- As you study, we suggest using this book as a notebook to jot down facts that you find particularly tricky or hard to remember. Having such **a personal and central database** for review can be invaluable during the final days before the exam. For this purpose wide margins are provided.
- The diagrams and tables in this book are very high yield. They are most useful if you can reproduce them on demand. Take advantage of active learning by re-drawing key diagrams and tables from memory. After you memorize some basic diagrams, many facts and pathways in biochemistry, physiology, and microbiology become easier to learn.
- During the last few days before the test, review each section in *Crashing the Boards* to make sure you do not lose easy points.

Test Taking Strategies

- Make sure you answer all questions. **There is no penalty for guessing.**
- To ensure that you finish the booklet, spend the first 30 seconds to write out a timeline. If the test starts at 1:05 PM, then write on the inside cover:

Time	Questions finished
1:35	30
2:05	60
2:35	90
3:05	120
3:35	150
4:05	End of exam

This pacing is particularly important for the first exam booklet, because many students fail to complete it.

- Difficult questions may yield to educated guessing algorithms. Is there something you have overlooked? Which answers can you eliminate? Is one answer significantly different from the others? Is one answer longer or more specific than the others?
- Fill in your answers in batches. A good batch size is one exam page or about six to ten questions. This technique saves time and reduces errors.
- There will be a few absurd questions on the exam. Many are experimental and will not be scored. Use them to save time. Circle the question in the test booklet, fill in your favorite letter, and move on. Check the question when you check your answers to make sure you did not overlook something obvious.
- If there is a picture, read the question first.

Avoiding Stupid Errors

- Read each question and answer carefully. No kidding. Careless errors can cost you many easily gettable points. The exam is long, and it is common to become lazy as time wears on. Remember, if you miss the word "not," you get the question wrong.
- Stick with your original choice unless you have a **good** reason for switching.
- In match lists, answers are rarely correct twice. Do not repeat an answer unless you are sure it is correct.
- **Do not despair if all the questions seem hard.** Remember that the average score on the USMLE Step 1 is about 65%. In most classes, this would be a flunking grade! In other words, you should expect to do far worse on the Boards percentage-wise than you have on almost every other test you've taken in your life.

Failing

Most students worry about failing both before and after taking the exam. The good news is that about 92% of first-time United States and Canadian examinees pass the USMLE Step 1 exam. The overall pass rate runs around 89%.

Failing the exam can be quite a blow. If the score seems wrong, the examinee may want to request a rescoring of his or her exam. The test center will recheck the scores by hand if it receives a written request and a fee is paid.

If a student fails, the first question to ask once the shock and disappointment wear off somewhat is when to retake the test. Many schools require passage of Step 1 to advance to the clinical years. Even more require passage for graduation. Students who fail the June exam are given two weeks or so after the scores are mailed to register for the September exam.

The student should consider carefully why he or she failed. As with a first attempt at the exam, future attempts should allow adequate study time, focus on high-yield topics, and employ effective study techniques. The performance profile sent out with the scores is the best way to identify areas of weakness. However, all high-yield subjects should be reviewed.

A Strategy for the Test Days

The day before   The day before the exam is a time for brief review and relaxation. Try to avoid studying new material. Unlike almost every other test you have taken in your life, last-minute overnight cramming will not pay off well. We suggest doing something fun in the evening. Obviously, drinking a lot of alcohol or caffeine is a bad idea.

Gather your supplies   Make sure you have everything you'll need for the exam. Know how to get to the test center and have reliable transportation, double check that you have your admission ticket and a valid photo ID, and make sure you have an eraser that works really well (rather than an old dried-up one that smudges) and a couple of #2 pencils (optional). Many also advise bringing a jacket, watch, analgesia, earplugs, and perhaps some food. Test conditions are rarely ideal. The air conditioner may be locked on, the clocks may be hard to see, or the building may be testing fire alarms all day.

The night before   The evening before the exam, the best thing you can do for yourself is to get a good night's sleep. However, even if you cannot sleep at all, we strongly suggest you still take the exam. It simply will not hurt you that much. Some students use sleeping aids such as diphenhydramine. (We'd say Benadryl, but on the Boards all drug names are generic!) Whatever you do, avoid anything you haven't taken before, and do not increase the dose.

Exam days　On the morning of the exam, be smart with what you eat and drink. Bathroom runs during the exam will be conducted one-at-a-time with an escort. No extra time will be given, even if you had two double espressos. Likewise for lunch, eat conservatively. Avoid eating a big meal that may make you sleepy or give you heartburn.

In between exam days, if you feel up to it, look up answers to some of the questions you did not know. The effort is high yield. Many Board exams appear to have themes that persist to the second day. Moreover, it is not uncommon to see questions repeated verbatim. One of us got the exact same question three times. (The answer is, of course, highlighted in this book.) If you are tired, go to bed early.

Don't forget your admission ticket, photo ID, jacket, and so on the next morning.

Best of luck on the exam!

Microbiology

CHAPTER 2

_____ **Coach's Tips**

- The bacterial cell wall, basic distinctions between bacteria, and bacterial virulence factors are important.
- Bacterial toxins are particularly popular.
- Antibiotics are popular. Mechanisms of action, major side effects, and major drug interactions are important. Bug coverage is not important.
- There will be several virology questions, but few questions on virus structures.
- Human immunodeficiency virus (HIV) is high yield.
- Viral enzymes are high yield.
- There will be a few questions on mycology and parasitology.

Bacteriology

_____ **Epidemiology**

- ***Streptococcus pneumoniae, Haemophilus influenzae,* and *Neisseria meningitidis*** are the important encapsulated organisms.
  - They are the top three causes of **bacterial meningitis.**
  - They are the top three infections that have **increased incidence** after **splenectomy.**
  - *N. meningitidis* is encapsulated, but *Neisseria gonorrhoeae* is not.
- **Meningitis time scale**

Age	*Organism*
0–2 months	*Escherichia coli* > Group B *Streptococcus*
3 months–21 years	*N. meningitidis* > *S. pneumoniae*
> 21 years	*S. pneumoniae*
Outbreaks	*N. meningitidis*

- **Epiglottitis** no longer has a classic cause thanks to the *H. influenzae* type b (Hib) vaccine. If asked for the #1 causative organism, the question is old and you should choose *H. influenzae*.
- **Live viral vaccines** include MMR (measles, mumps, rubella), varicella, and polio. Sabin is live.

Mnemonic: *"Sal**k** is **k**illed."*

Bacterial Cell Walls

Gram-positive cell wall

Gram-positive cell walls have **teichoic acid** and a thick peptidoglycan wall.

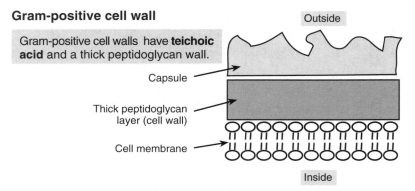

Outside

Capsule

Thick peptidoglycan layer (cell wall)

Cell membrane

Inside

Gram-negative cell wall

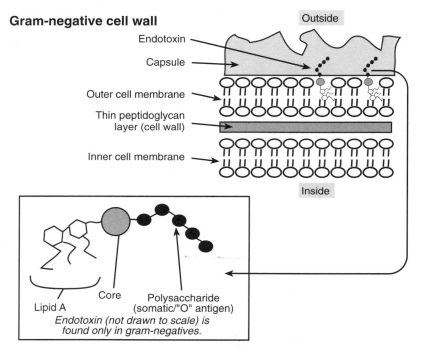

Outside

Endotoxin

Capsule

Outer cell membrane

Thin peptidoglycan layer (cell wall)

Inner cell membrane

Inside

Lipid A

Core

Polysaccharide (somatic/"O" antigen)

Endotoxin (not drawn to scale) is found only in gram-negatives.

General cell wall facts
- All capsules are **antiphagocytic**.
- All capsules are made of polysaccharides. The exception is the gram-negative *Bacillus*, which has D-glutamate.
- Both gram-positives and gram-negatives have **porins**, which are small holes in the cell wall that allow small hydrophilic molecules into the cell.
- *Mycoplasma* lacks a cell wall, so antibiotics directed against cell walls do not affect it.
- *Mycobacteria*, like fungi, have mycolic acids in their cell membrane.

Virulence Factors

These are mostly protein molecules that mediate adherence and hinder phagocytosis.

Adherence
- M protein: *Streptococcus* species
- Pili: *N. gonorrhoeae, E. coli,* Group A *Streptococcus*
- Protein II: *N. gonorrhoeae*

Antiphagocytic
- Capsule: *S. pneumoniae, H. influenzae,* **and** *N. meningitidis* are the important ones.
- Intracellular survival: *Mycobacteria, Listeria,* and *Legionella* survive in cells by inhibiting the fusion of lysosomes with phagosomes.
- Motility: *Proteus* and *Salmonella*

Anti-opsonization
- Immunoglobulin A (IgA) protease: *S. pneumoniae, H. influenzae, N. meningitidis,* and *N. gonorrhoeae*
- H-antigen (flagella): Some *Salmonella* species can **phase-shift** to evade the immune response

Unknown Mechanism
- Cord factor: *Mycobacterium tuberculosis*

Toxins

Endotoxin
- Is a lipopolysaccharide (especially **lipid A**) present **only in gram-negative bacteria**
- Is an **integral part of the outer membrane of the cell wall**
- Is not released from the cell
- Causes fever, hypotension, and shock

Exotoxins
- Are (glyco)proteins that **are released** locally or into the circulation

Diphtheria toxin
- The A subunit permanently inactivates elongation factor 2 (EF-2) by adenosine diphosphate (ADP)-ribosylation.

Bordetella pertussis toxins
- Stimulate adenylate cyclase by ADP-ribosylation
- Secrete adenylate cyclase, which has antiphagocytic action

Clostridium tetani (tetanospasmin)
- Blocks release of inhibitory neurotransmitter **glycine** in brain, causing extreme muscle spasm

Clostridium botulinum (botulinin)	• Blocks presynaptic release of acetylcholine
Clostridium difficile	• Exotoxin A: causes outpouring of fluid
	• Exotoxin B: cytotoxin; damages gut mucosa
	• ***C. difficile* test:** assays for exotoxins in stool
Bacillus anthracis	• A single exotoxin with three components: adenylate cyclase edema factor, protective antigen, and lethal factor
Pseudomonas species	• Exotoxin A: inhibits eukaryotic protein synthesis by ADP-ribosylation of EF-2 (same as diphtheria)
Cholera toxin (choleragen)	• Stimulates adenylate cyclase by ADP-ribosylation
E. coli	• Heat-stable toxin: stimulates guanylate cyclase
	• Heat-labile toxin (like cholera toxin): stimulates adenylate cyclase by ADP-ribosylation
	• Verotoxin: inactivates protein synthesis by removing adenine from the 28S ribosomal RNA (rRNA) part of the 60S subunit of the human ribosome (***Shigella*** also has verotoxin)
Staphylococcus aureus toxins	• **TSST (toxic shock syndrome toxin):** a "**superantigen**" causing toxic shock; binds to class II major histocompatibility complex (MHC) proteins; induces interleukin-1 (IL-1) and IL-2
	• Protein A: antiphagocytic; binds to Fc portion of IgG, preventing the binding of complement
	• Coagulase: accelerates clotting, which may protect from phagocytosis
	• Many other toxins
Streptococcus pyogenes toxins (Group A *Streptococcus*)	• Streptolysin O: a hemolysin
	• Many other toxins

Basic Laboratory Differentiation

Organisms That Do Not Gram Stain

- *Rickettsiae* are intracellular.
- *Chlamydia* are intracellular and sometimes cause **cytoplasmic inclusions.**

- *Mycobacteria* are intracellular, but can be seen on acid-fast carbol-fuchsin stain.
- *Spirochetes* (*Treponema, Borrelia, Leptospira*) are too thin to be seen on Gram stain but can be seen by darkfield.
- *Mycoplasma* have no cell wall (they only have a **plasma** membrane), so they do not stain.

Additional Tidbits
- *H. influenzae* and *N. meningitidis* grow *only* on cooked blood (chocolate agar). The other gram-negative rods grow on chocolate agar *and* uncooked blood puree. *Mnemonic: How Nice! Chocolate!*
- Urease cleaves urea to a CO_2 and two NH_3. The NH_3 combines with H^+ to form NH_4^+, thus increasing the pH.
- *Proteus* causes urinary tract infections.
- *Helicobacter pylori* causes gastrointestinal (GI) ulcers (increased pH allows *H. pylori* to survive).
- The sulfur producers (H_2S gas) are *Proteus* and *Salmonella*.

Antibiotics

Coach's Hint: *In general, mechanism of action and side effects are important, but coverage is not. Nevertheless, here we list some important coverage facts.*

Important Bacteria Coverage Points
- Erythromycin is the drug of choice for *Mycoplasma, Chlamydia, Legionella,* and *Bordetella* (the causes of "atypical" pneumonia).
- Metronidazole and *oral* vancomycin are used for pseudomembranous colitis. Vancomycin is not absorbed by the GI tract.
- Penicillin V is absorbed orally much better than penicillin G.
- Metronidazole kills anaerobes and protozoa.
- Tetracycline is the drug of choice for *Rickettsia*.
- Among cephalosporins, only third and fourth generation drugs reliably penetrate the blood-brain barrier.
- First generation cephalosporins cover gram-positives best. Third and fourth generation cephalosporins cover gram-negatives best.

Antibiotic Enhancer	Used With	Mechanism
Clavulanic acid, sulbactam	Penicillins	β-Lactamase inhibitors
Probenecid (a gout drug)	Penicillins	Decreases renal clearance
Cilastatin	Imipenem	Inhibits renal metabolism

Gram-Negative Bacteria

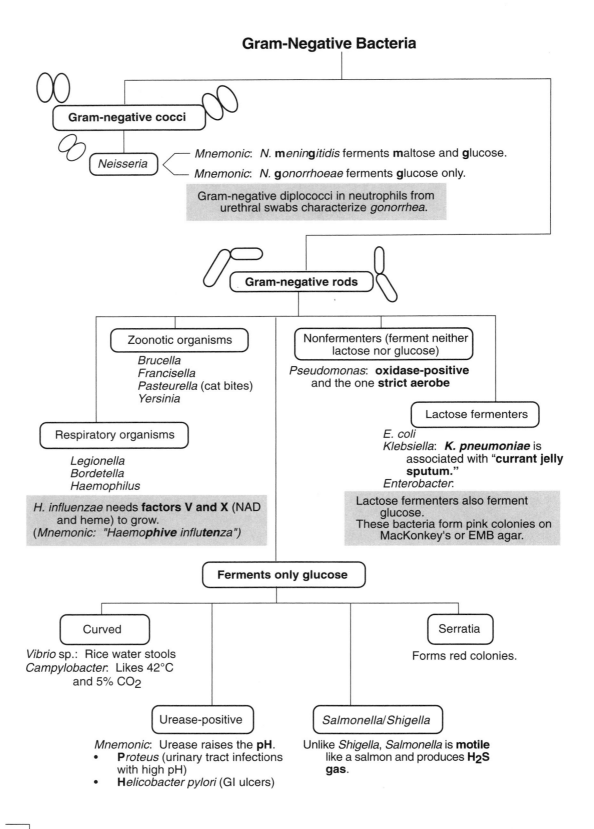

Gram-negative cocci

Neisseria

Mnemonic: *N.* **m**enin**g**itidis ferments **m**altose and **g**lucose.
Mnemonic: *N.* **g**onorrhoeae ferments **g**lucose only.

Gram-negative diplococci in neutrophils from urethral swabs characterize *gonorrhea*.

Gram-negative rods

Zoonotic organisms

Brucella
Francisella
Pasteurella (cat bites)
Yersinia

Respiratory organisms

Legionella
Bordetella
Haemophilus

H. influenzae needs **factors V and X** (NAD and heme) to grow.
(*Mnemonic*: "Haemo**phive influtenza**")

Nonfermenters (ferment neither lactose nor glucose)

Pseudomonas: **oxidase-positive** and the one **strict aerobe**

Lactose fermenters

E. coli
Klebsiella: **K. pneumoniae** is associated with "**currant jelly sputum.**"
Enterobacter.

Lactose fermenters also ferment glucose.
These bacteria form pink colonies on MacKonkey's or EMB agar.

Ferments only glucose

Curved

Vibrio sp.: Rice water stools
Campylobacter: Likes 42°C and 5% CO_2

Urease-positive

Mnemonic: Urease raises the **pH**.
- **P**roteus (urinary tract infections with high pH)
- **H**elicobacter pylori (GI ulcers)

Salmonella/Shigella

Unlike *Shigella*, *Salmonella* is **motile** like a salmon and produces **H_2S gas**.

Serratia

Forms red colonies.

Gram-Positive Bacteria

Mnemonic: Gram-positives are blue—think "B+")

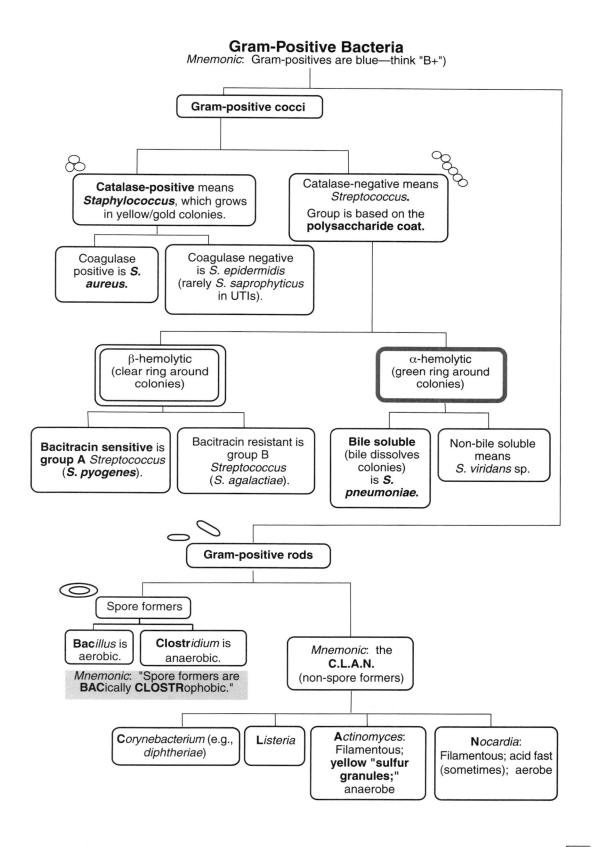

Gram-positive cocci

Catalase-positive means ***Staphylococcus***, which grows in yellow/gold colonies.

Catalase-negative means *Streptococcus*.

Group is based on the **polysaccharide coat.**

Coagulase positive is ***S. aureus.***

Coagulase negative is *S. epidermidis* (rarely *S. saprophyticus* in UTIs).

β-hemolytic (clear ring around colonies)

α-hemolytic (green ring around colonies)

Bacitracin sensitive is **group A** *Streptococcus* (***S. pyogenes***).

Bacitracin resistant is group B *Streptococcus* (*S. agalactiae*).

Bile soluble (bile dissolves colonies) is ***S. pneumoniae.***

Non-bile soluble means *S. viridans* sp.

Gram-positive rods

Spore formers

Bac*illus* is aerobic.

Clostr*idium* is anaerobic.

Mnemonic: "Spore formers are **BAC**ically **CLOSTR**ophobic."

Mnemonic: the **C.L.A.N.** (non-spore formers)

C*orynebacterium* (e.g., *diphtheriae*)

L*isteria*

A*ctinomyces*: Filamentous; **yellow "sulfur granules;"** anaerobe

N*ocardia*: Filamentous; acid fast (sometimes); aerobe

Antibiotic	Side Effects
Penicillins	Anaphylaxis; rash
Cephalosporins	Anaphylaxis; rash; among penicillin-allergics, 2%–10% are cephalosporin-allergic
Imipenem	Seizures
Vancomycin	Red man syndrome if infused quickly (tachycardia, flushing, kills kidneys, hypotension); hearing loss
Aminoglycosides	Hearing loss; **kidney damage**
Tetracyclines	Photosensitivity; causes yellow teeth and bad bones in children; **shouldn't be taken with antacids** or milk (prevents absorption)
Chloramphenicol	Dose-dependent aplastic anemia; **gray baby syndrome** (damages fetal heart and lungs)
Erythromycin	GI (nausea, diarrhea)
Clindamycin	**Pseudomembranous colitis** caused by *C. difficile;* treated with oral vancomycin or metronidazole
Fluoroquinolones	**Shouldn't be taken with antacids** or iron (divalent metals chelate the drug and prevent absorption); not given to children because it may cause arrest of growth plates by inhibiting cartilage synthesis
Rifampin	Turns body secretions (saliva, urine, sweat) red ("red-armpit"); hepatotoxic
Sulfonamides	Bone marrow depression; rash
Trimethoprim	Bone marrow suppression
Metronidazole	Causes disulfiram-like reaction with alcohol consumption
Amphotericin B	Very toxic—kills kidneys, liver, brain

Isoniazid

- Isoniazid is used to treat a positive tuberculin skin test in a healthy individual.
- Isoniazid causes **peripheral neuropathy** and age-related **hepatitis.**
- Pyridoxine (**vitamin B$_6$**) helps to prevent peripheral neuropathy.

Miscellaneous

- Almost all antibiotic resistance is transmitted by **plasmids via conjugation.**
- Gut and peritoneal abscesses are often due to *Bacteroides.*
- *H. pylori* is implicated in gastric and duodenal ulcers. It protects

Antibiotic Mechanisms

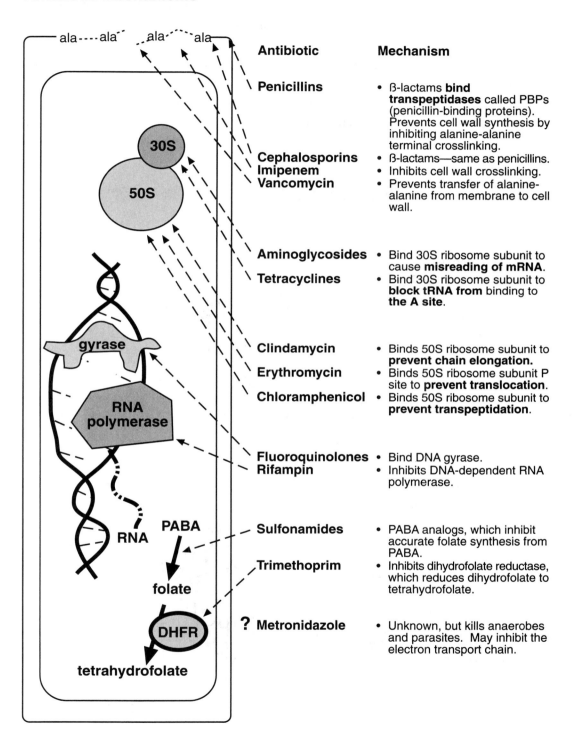

Antibiotic	Mechanism
Penicillins	• ß-lactams **bind transpeptidases** called PBPs (penicillin-binding proteins). Prevents cell wall synthesis by inhibiting alanine-alanine terminal crosslinking.
Cephalosporins **Imipenem** **Vancomycin**	• ß-lactams—same as penicillins. • Inhibits cell wall crosslinking. • Prevents transfer of alanine-alanine from membrane to cell wall.
Aminoglycosides **Tetracyclines**	• Bind 30S ribosome subunit to cause **misreading of mRNA.** • Bind 30S ribosome subunit to **block tRNA from** binding to **the A site.**
Clindamycin **Erythromycin** **Chloramphenicol**	• Binds 50S ribosome subunit to **prevent chain elongation.** • Binds 50S ribosome subunit P site to **prevent translocation.** • Binds 50S ribosome subunit to **prevent transpeptidation.**
Fluoroquinolones **Rifampin**	• Bind DNA gyrase. • Inhibits DNA-dependent RNA polymerase.
Sulfonamides **Trimethoprim**	• PABA analogs, which inhibit accurate folate synthesis from PABA. • Inhibits dihydrofolate reductase, which reduces dihydrofolate to tetrahydrofolate.
? Metronidazole	• Unknown, but kills anaerobes and parasites. May inhibit the electron transport chain.

itself from gastric acid by producing **urease.** *H. pylori* can be eradicated by antibiotics combined with **bismuth** agents.

- *Vibrio cholerae* binds to mucous membranes by secreting an **enzyme that dissolves mucus.**

Rickettsiae
- Lyme disease: *Borrelia burgdorferi*, transmitted by the *Ixodes* deer tick
- Rocky Mountain spotted fever: *Rickettsia rickettsii*
- Q fever: *Coxiella burnetii*

Mycology

Mycoses

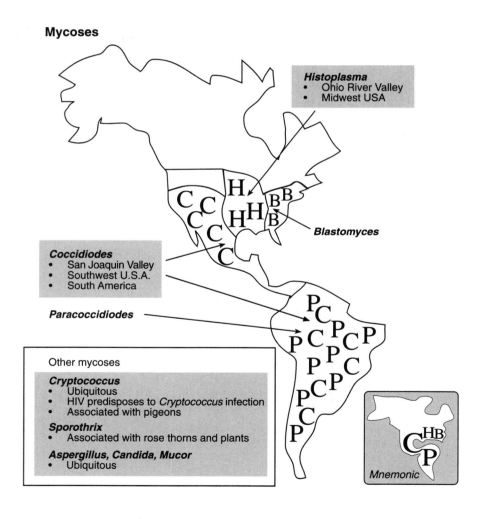

Histoplasma
- Ohio River Valley
- Midwest USA

Blastomyces

Coccidiodes
- San Joaquin Valley
- Southwest U.S.A.
- South America

Paracoccidiodes

Other mycoses

Cryptococcus
- Ubiquitous
- HIV predisposes to *Cryptococcus* infection
- Associated with pigeons

Sporothrix
- Associated with rose thorns and plants

Aspergillus, Candida, Mucor
- Ubiquitous

Mnemonic

Parasitology

Malaria
- Malaria kills a million people a year. It is the #1 fatal infection worldwide.
- Female *Anopheles* **mosquitoes** transmit the *Plasmodium,* which go to the **liver.**
- Every three days or so, parasites are released into the blood, causing hemolysis.
- Hemolysis causes **periodic bouts of high fever,** drenching sweats, vomiting, and headache. Hemorrhage, brain necrosis, and kidney damage can result, especially with *Plasmodium falciparum.*
- Sickle cell trait is protective against malaria.

Schistosoma
- *Schistosoma* alternate between human and freshwater snail hosts.
- Early infection can cause fever, diarrhea, lymphadenopathy, and eosinophilia.
- *Schistosoma mansoni* (Africa, Latin America) and *Schistosoma japonicum* (Asia) invade the gut veins. They cause cirrhosis, **portal hypertension,** and splenomegaly. Patients can die from ruptured esophageal varices.
- *Schistosoma haematobium* (Africa, Middle East) invade the veins, draining the urinary bladder. It causes hematuria and **bladder carcinoma.**

Giardia
- *Giardia lamblia* is a protozoa that lives in humans and animals.
- It causes persistent nonbloody diarrhea and nausea without fever.
- It is common in hikers who drink untreated water and in male homosexuals.
- Transmission is fecal–oral.

Miscellaneous
- Barefoot children get *Strongyloides* and hookworm.
- Pinworms (*Enterobius vermicularis*) are the #1 cause of anal itching in children in the United States.

Virology

Coach's hint: If **giant cells** are involved, think **measles, herpes,** or **respiratory syncytial virus (RSV).**

RNA Viruses

- **Reovirus is double-stranded.** All other RNA viruses are single-stranded.
- The **influenza virus** has eight genome segments. Co-infection of a cell by two different influenza strains may lead to genome **reassortment,** causing a **genetic shift.** Yearly influenza vaccines address genetic shifts.
- Retrovirus and reovirus are also segmented.

DNA Viruses

Important General Points

Mnemonic:

- **Parvovirus is the only single-stranded DNA virus.**
  "part of a virus"
- These are listed in order of increasing size: parvovirus is the smallest and poxvirus the largest.

Nonenveloped DNA Viruses

Family	DNA Strand Orientation	Important Pathogens
Parvovirus	SS	B19—fifth disease with "slapped cheek" rash
Papovavirus	DS, circular, supercoiled	HPV—warts
Adenovirus	DS, linear	Adenovirus

DS = double-stranded; HPV = human papillomavirus; SS = single-stranded.

Enveloped DNA Viruses

Family	DNA Strand Orientation	Important Pathogens
Hepadnavirus	DS, incompletely circular	Hepatitis B
Herpesvirus	DS, linear	HSV, VZV, CMV, EBV
Poxvirus	DS, linear	Smallpox (vaccinia)

CMV = cytomegalovirus; EBV = Epstein-Barr virus; HSV = herpes simplex virus; VZV = varicella-zoster virus.

- **HPVs** tend to cause benign tumors of squamous cells. There are at least 60 serotypes.
  - ○ HPV 6, 11—genital warts
  - ○ HPV 16, 18—carcinoma of the cervix and penis
- Adenovirus infects mucosal epithelia of the respiratory tract, GI tract, and conjunctiva.
- After primary infection, herpesviruses typically lie dormant in nerve cell bodies. Infection may recur years later.

Virus	Primary Infection	Latency Site	Recurrent Infection
HSV-1	Gingivostomatitis	Cranial sensory nerve ganglia (CN V)	Herpes labialis, encephalitis
HSV-2	Genital herpes	Sensory ganglia	Genital herpes
VZV	Varicella (chickenpox)	Sensory ganglia	Zoster (shingles)
EBV	**Mononucleosis**	B lymphocytes	Usually none

- HSV-1 typically occurs above the neck, HSV-2 below the waist.
- EBV causes infectious mononucleosis. Blood smears show **atypical lymphocytes.** The serum is **heterophil positive.**
- CMV may cause congenital malformations (deafness, microcephaly, seizures, mental retardation).
- The **ToRCH** organisms are important causes of **congenital malformations** and **neonatal infections.**

Toxoplasmosis
Rubella
Cytomegalovirus
Herpes simplex 2

Human Immunodeficiency Virus (HIV)

*HIV is the **retrovirus** responsible for the acquired immune deficiency syndrome (AIDS). It is the most tested virus on the USMLE Step 1.*

Important Retrovirus Facts	• It is an **RNA** virus.

Important Retrovirus Facts

- It is an **RNA** virus.
- It carries **reverse transcriptase,** an RNA-dependent DNA polymerase that makes double-stranded DNA.
- It is the **only known diploid virus.** Each virion carries two identical single-stranded positive-polarity RNA molecules.

Pathophysiology and Disease Specifics

- HIV is spread by sexual contact, through transfusions with infected blood, and transplacentally.
- Homosexual males, intravenous (IV) drug users, and hemophiliacs were the initial high risk groups.
- Using condoms and not sharing needles reduce transmission.
- The surface protein **gp120 binds to CD4 to initiate infection.**
- HIV infects and kills **helper T cells,** which express the protein **CD4.**
- HIV also infects other CD4⁺ cells, such as macrophages and monocytes.
- Loss of helper T cells causes **suppression of cell mediated immunity.**
- Two to four weeks after infection, a mononucleosis-like syndrome occurs. A latent period of 1–10 years then ensues.
- **AIDS is defined by HIV infection with a helper T cell count less than 200/mm³ or the presence of one or more AIDS-related infections and neoplasms with or without a low T cell count.**
- The top two manifestations of AIDS are *Pneumocystis pneumonia* and **Kaposi's sarcoma.**
- **Non-Hodgkins lymphoma** is also important.
- Opportunistic infections increase as the T cell count drops. These include **tuberculosis,** herpes simplex, herpes zoster, CMV, *Candida* (especially oral thrush), cryptococcal meningitis, and toxoplasmosis.

Drug Therapy for HIV

- Antiretroviral drugs prolong survival but do not cure.
- HIV develops resistance quickly to any of these agents if single drugs are used, so they are prescribed in combination.

Nucleoside reverse transcriptase inhibitors

- Nucleoside reverse transcriptase inhibitors inhibit HIV reverse transcriptase by acting as DNA chain terminators. For example, AZT (zidovudine, azidothymidine) is a thymidine analog. Because AZT has

Structure of the Human Immunodeficiency Virus

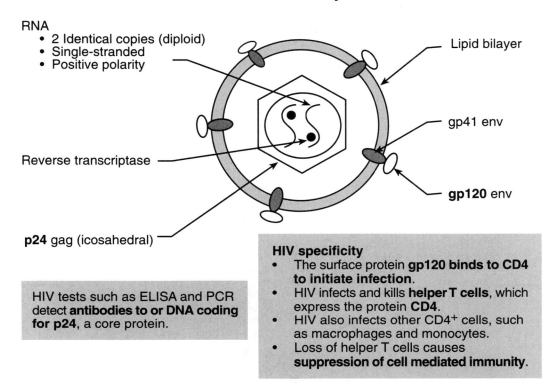

RNA
- 2 Identical copies (diploid)
- Single-stranded
- Positive polarity

Lipid bilayer

gp41 env

Reverse transcriptase

gp120 env

p24 gag (icosahedral)

HIV tests such as ELISA and PCR detect **antibodies to or DNA coding for p24**, a core protein.

HIV specificity
- The surface protein **gp120 binds to CD4 to initiate infection**.
- HIV infects and kills **helper T cells**, which express the protein **CD4**.
- HIV also infects other CD4+ cells, such as macrophages and monocytes.
- Loss of helper T cells causes **suppression of cell mediated immunity**.

no 3′ phosphate group, no bases can be added after it. **Viral thymidine kinase** uses AZT much more efficiently than does human thymidine kinase. Thus, AZT slows viral DNA replication.

Drug	Side Effects
Zidovudine (AZT)	**GI upset,** anemia
Stavudine (d4T)	Peripheral neuropathy, GI upset
Zalcitabine (ddC)	Peripheral neuropathy, GI upset, pancreatitis
Didanosine (ddI)	Peripheral neuropathy, GI upset, pancreatitis
Lamivudine (3TC)	Rash

Protease inhibitors
- Protease inhibitors prevent cleavage of the HIV proteins required for viral replication. The uncleaved proteins do not work.

Drug	Side Effects	Notes
Indinavir	**Kidney stones**	
Ritonavir	Nausea and diarrhea	Inhibits P-450 system
Saquinavir	Nausea	Metabolized by P-450 system

Inhibitory mechanisms of Antiviral Drugs

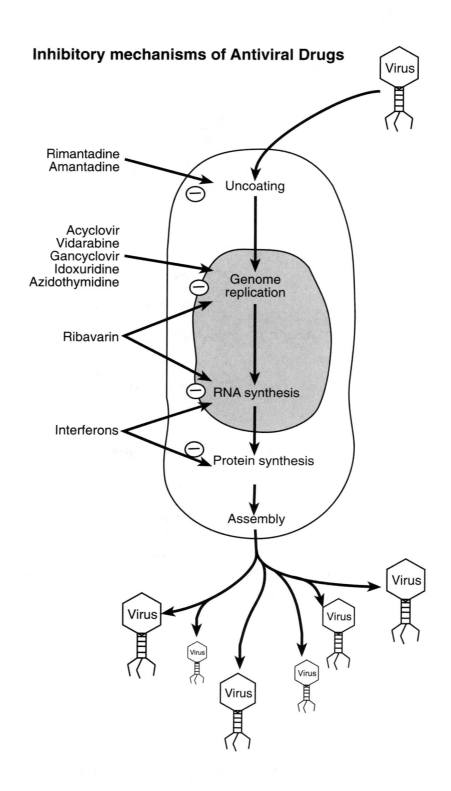

Nonnucleoside reverse
transcriptase inhibitors

- Nonnucleoside reverse transcriptase inhibitors include nevirapine and delavirdine. They cause rashes.

Other Antiviral Drugs

Inhibitors of Early Events

- Amantadine prevents viral uncoating of influenza A.

Inhibitors of Viral Nucleic Acid Synthesis

- Nucleoside and nucleotide analogs preferentially terminate viral DNA chains.
- **Viral nucleoside kinases often catalyze the phosphorylation of these drugs into the triphosphate form.**

Drug	Structural Modification	Organisms
Acyclovir	Guanine analog	HSV, VZV
Ganciclovir	Guanine analog	CMV
Vidarabine (AraA)	Adenosine analog	HSV-1
Ribavirin	Guanosine analog	RSV

Inhibitors of Viral Protein Synthesis

- Interferons

Immunology

CHAPTER 3

Coach's Tips

_____

- Basic mechanisms of B cell and T cell activation are important.
- Immunoglobulin (Ig) classes and major histocompatibility complex (MHC) classes are important.
- Several questions will ask about infant immune responses to bacteria and vaccines.
- Immune deficiency syndromes such as acquired immune deficiency syndrome (AIDS), severe combined immunodeficiency, and Ché-diak-Higashi are high yield.

Basic Immunology

_____

- **CD8$^+$** cells have T cell receptors that respond to **MHC I** molecules that have bound epitopes. These epitopes come from **inside** the cell. CD8$^+$ T cells may also be suppresser T cells.
- **CD4$^+$** cells respond to **MHC II** bound to epitopes derived from antibody binding or phagocytosis.
- The ratio of CD4$^+$ to CD8$^+$ cells is 2:1 in a healthy person.
- The fetus makes IgM, but the amount is **small relative to the amount of IgG that the fetus receives from the mother** across the placenta. Maternal IgG in the newborn works for approximately 6 months.
- The T cell receptor (TCR) specifically recognizes antigen only in conjunction with self MHC molecules. However, TCRs may be activated nonspecifically by non-self MHC molecules.
- Superantigens **nonspecifically** link TCRs to MHC molecules, thus activating T cells **without internal processing.** Superantigens may play a role in T cell maturation (good) and in the pathogenesis of toxic shock syndrome and other infections (bad).
- Rejection of transplanted organs is based on MHC II (especially the DR locus), T helper cells, and cytotoxic T cells.
- CD5 is a marker found in fetal B cells and is an important marker in **chronic lymphocytic leukemia (CLL).**

Quick Immunoglobulin Facts

IgM
- The main Ig in the primary response
- IgM is a pentamer, has the highest binding avidity of all antibodies, and has a J chain.

IgA
- The secretory Ig
- IgA is found wherever the outside meets the inside [tears, saliva, **breast milk,** GI tract, genitourinary (GU) tract].
- IgA is usually a **dimer,** has a **J chain,** and has a **secretory component** that prevents degradation in the GI tract.

IgE
- The main Ig in allergic responses
- IgE is found on the surface of basophils and mast cells.
- IgE is **not found on eosinophils.**

IgG
- The main Ig involved in the amnestic (secondary) response
- IgG and C3b (a component of complement) are the only substances that can **opsonize.**
- IgG is also the only Ig that crosses the placenta.

IgD
- IgD is found on the surface of mature B cells (not plasma cells).
- IgD and IgM are **simultaneously** produced by B cells by **alternative splicing.**

Antibody Response
- The primary antibody response (IgM) occurs in 7 to 10 days. Later during the same exposure, IgG levels also rise.
- On re-exposure, the secondary (amnestic) response (IgG) occurs in 3 to 5 days with higher levels of antibody, higher antibody avidity (binding strength), and longer antibody response.
- T cell **independent** antibody responses are triggered by repeating nonprotein antigens such as endotoxins and many bacterial **polysaccharides.** They **nonspecifically** activate B cells and elicit IgM only. Because there is no T cell "help," there is no isotype switching.

Cytokines

Cytokine	Made By	Functions
IL-1	Macrophages	**Activates helper T cells,** causes fever (the "endogenous pyrogen")
IL-2	Helper T cells	Stimulates **T cell growth**
IL-4	Helper T cells	B cell **growth,** Ig class switch to IgA
IL-5	Helper T cells	B cell **differentiation** into plasma cells, Ig class switch to IgE
IFNγ	Most T cells	Acts on macrophages, NK cells, and PMNs to stimulate phagocytosis
TNFα	Macrophages	Activates PMNs, mediates septic shock, causes necrosis of tumors, also called cachectin

IFN = interferon; IL = interleukin; NK = natural killer; PMNs = polymorphonuclear nucleocytes; TNF = tumor necrosis factor.

- The anaphylatoxins C3a, C4a, and especially C5a trigger mast cell degranulation.
- C5a attracts neutrophils.
- Lack of late components of complement (C5–C8) predisposes to *Neisseria* bacteremia.
- Deficiency of C3 predisposes to pyogenic bacterial infections (*Staphylococcus aureus*).
- The membrane attack complex consists of C5b–C9.

Pediatric Immunology

Type of Immunity	Status in Infants
Cell-mediated (T cells)	Well developed
Phagocytosis/complement	Roughly halved until 6 months old
	Susceptible to severe systemic bacterial infection until 6 months old
Antibodies (B cells)	**No response to most polysaccharide antigens until 2 years old**
	Response to protein antigens well developed
	Maternal IgG protective until 6 months old
	Infants produce IgG, but not enough
Antiviral	**Maternal IgG protective until 6 months old**
	Weak antiviral immunity from 6 months to 5 years old, leading to many viral infections.

Immunodeficiency Syndromes

IgA deficiency
- Selective IgA deficiency is the #1 primary immunodeficiency disorder.
- Some patients get recurrent sinusitis, pneumonia, and *Giardia* infections.
- IgG and IgM are normal.

X-linked
agammaglobulinemia **B cells are virtually absent,** so all immunoglobulins are decreased.

- Recurrent pyogenic infections begin around six months of age, when maternal antibodies decline.

Wiskott-Aldrich
- An X-linked deficiency in humoral and cellular immunity leads to eczema, thrombocytopenia, and recurrent bacterial infections.
- IgM is low, reducing antibacterial immunity.

DiGeorge syndrome (thymic dysplasia)
- The 3rd and 4th pharyngeal pouches fail to develop.
- The thymus, parathyroid glands, and portions of the aortic arch are affected, causing **extreme T cell deficiency, tetany** from hypocalcemia, and sometimes truncus arteriosus.
- T cell deficiency leads to viral, fungal, protozoal, and intracellular bacterial infections.
- B cell and immunoglobulin function are completely normal.

Severe combined immunodeficiency
- It is usually X-linked.
- Both B cells and T cells are absent.
- Most patients lack antibody-dependent cell toxicity and NK cell function.
- **Adenosine deaminase is deficient** in 20%.
- Patients die of various infections.

Chronic granulomatous disease
- It is usually X-linked.
- **Lack of reduced nicotinamide adenine dinucleotide phosphate (NADPH) oxidase activity** favors fungi and catalase-producing organisms like *Staphylococcus.*
- Recurrent *Staphylococcus* infections are typical.

Chédiak-Higashi
- An autosomal recessive defect in neutrophil and NK cell function leads to giant, **nonfunctional lysosomes.**
- Recurrent *Staphylococcus* and *Streptococcus* sinusitis and pneumonia are typical.

Chronic mucocutaneous candidiasis
- Patients have a specific T cell defect for *Candida albicans.*

Hereditary angioedema
- It is an autosomal dominant defect in C1 esterase inhibitor.
- Organ edema can be fatal.

Pharmacology

CHAPTER 4

Joy Y. Wu

_____ **Coach's Tips**

- **If the physiology is known, the Board authors like it.** Try to learn the drugs while you learn the related topics. For example, study heart drugs and cardiac physiology at the same time. This both aids memory and directs learning toward high-yield drugs.
- Mechanisms of drug **actions, side effects, and toxicities** are most important. The test focuses on side effects that either illustrate points of physiology or are life-threatening.
- Cardiovascular, central nervous system (CNS), adrenergic, and cholinergic drugs are emphasized. In particular, each question on adrenergic and cholinergic drugs typically requires in-depth knowledge of several drugs. Consequently, these sections are high yield *if* they are memorized in detail.
- All drug names are **generic.** Questions will ask about fluoxetine, not Prozac.
- Drug dosages are almost never tested.
- Questions rarely ask which antibiotic kills which microorganism.
- Questions rarely ask which chemotherapy agent is used for which neoplasm.

_____ **Pharmacokinetics Facts**

Half-Life
- **Half-life** comes in two forms.
  - *(1)* The **distribution half-life** is the time it takes for 50% of the drug to redistribute from the blood plasma to fat, the brain, and other tissues.
  - *(2)* The **elimination half-life** is the time it takes to remove 50% of the drug from the body.
- With continuous infusion, it takes **four or five half-lives** to reach steady-state plasma concentrations.
- Increasing the rate of infusion **will not shorten the time it takes to reach steady state.** It still takes four to five half-lives.

Affinity, Efficacy, and Potency
- **Affinity** refers to the strength of binding of a drug to its receptor. Affinity is measured by the dissociation constant (K_d). K_d is the concentration of drug required to achieve 50% occupancy of its receptors.
- **Efficacy** is the maximum effect achievable with the drug at any concentration.
- **Potency** is the amount of drug needed to achieve 50% of maximum effect.
- For Board purposes, **affinity has nothing to do with potency or efficacy.**

Metabolism
- Drug metabolism makes drugs more polar to enhance elimination. Most metabolism occurs in the **liver.**
- Phase 1 reactions are nonsynthetic. Drugs are oxidized and reduced, mainly in the cytochrome P-450 system.
- Phase 2 reactions are synthetic. Polar groups such as acetyls are added. All conjugations and acetylations are phase 2.
- Several drugs **induce the cytochrome P-450 system,** thus increasing the rate of drug metabolism. **Phenobarbital** and **alcohol** are the classic examples. In contrast, **cimetidine inhibits** the P-450 system.

Clearance
- Drug clearance is the volume of blood completely cleared of drug in a given time (ml/minute or liters/day). Be prepared to calculate clearance by one of the following two equations.

$$\text{Clearance = Elimination rate / Drug concentration}$$

  - Where:
    - Elimination rate is the amount of drug removed per unit time, commonly expressed in mg/hr.
    - Drug concentration is normally the plasma concentration.

Or,
$$\text{Clearance} = k \times V_d$$

  - Where:
    - k is the elimination rate constant (k will be given to you, although it may not be obvious).
    - V_d is the apparent volume of distribution. It is the theoretical volume of plasma required to contain a dose if the dose were evenly distributed at plasma concentration levels.
- *Example:* If the plasma concentration is 1 mg/liter after 20 mg of a drug is given, then V_d = 20 mg/1 mg/liter, or 20 liters.

Other
- Loading dose = $V_d \times$ desired plasma concentration
- Maintenance dose = plasma level $\times$ clearance

Adrenergic Drugs

- For almost all of these drugs, **the receptor-mediated effects and the "side effects" are the same thing.** The hard questions will give tracings of heart rate, blood pressure, and smooth muscle tension (a.k.a. bronchiole or artery wall tension) and ask which drug was given at which point.

Adrenergic Receptors

α_1	α_2	β_1	β_2
Vasoconstricts	Reduces CNS sympathetics	Increases heart rate and contractility	Bronchodilates Vasodilates
Constipates	Shuts off insulin	Stimulates lipolysis	Relaxes the uterus

β *mnemonic:* **One heart(β_1), two lungs(β_2).**

Adrenergic Agonists

Agonist	*Receptor*	*Effects*
Phenylephrine	α_1 only	Vasoconstriction, **reflex bradycardia,** BP up
Norepinephrine	Intense α_1; weak $\beta_1 > \beta_2$	Vasoconstriction, **reflex bradycardia,** BP up
Amphetamine	Releases norepinephrine	Vasoconstriction, **reflex bradycardia,** BP up
Ephedrine	Releases norepinephrine > epinephrine	Vasoconstriction, HR up, BP up
Epinephrine	Strong α_1, β_1; moderate β_2	Vasoconstriction, HR up, BP up
Isoproterenol	Strong β_1, β_2	Vasodilation, HR up, BP down (strong!)
Dobutamine	Moderate $\beta_1 > \beta_2$	Vasodilation, HR up
Metaproterenol	Mainly β_2	Vasodilation, HR can go up (a β_1 effect)
Dopamine	Dopamine $> \beta_1$	**Shunts blood to kidneys,** HR up
Albuterol	Mainly β_2	**Bronchodilation,** HR can go up (β_1)
Terbutaline	Mainly β_2	**Relaxes uterus** to treat premature labor

BP = blood pressure; HR = heart rate.

• Dopamine in high doses will cause vasoconstriction because of α agonism.

• α Agonists raise systemic vascular resistance by constricting blood vessels. The body then reduces cardiac output to keep blood pressure from skyrocketing (BP = CO × SVR). Cardiac output is reduced by slowing heart rate, hence the term **reflex bradycardia.**

Adrenergic Antagonists

Antagonist	Receptor	Effects
Phenoxybenzamine	α_1, α_2	Vasodilation, BP way down
Phentolamine	α_1, α_2	Vasodilation, BP way down
Prazosin	α_1	Vasodilation, BP down
Propranolol	β_1, β_2	BP down, HR down, contractility down, O$_2$ demand down, **β_2 effects cause bronchoconstriction and impair glucose control**
Atenolol	β_1 selective	BP down, HR down, contractility down, O$_2$ demand down
Metoprolol	β_1 selective	BP down, HR down, contractility down, O$_2$ demand down

Key points • If it ends in **-*lol*** it is a β **blocker.** If it ends in -rol or -nol, it is a β agonist.

• **Propranolol is not used in asthmatics.** Its β_2 antagonism causes bronchoconstriction.

• Propranolol is used for migraine prophylaxis.

• Phenoxybenzamine is used to treat pheochromocytoma before surgery.

Presynaptic Adrenergic Blockers

Drug	Mechanism	Effects
Reserpine	Depletes catecholamines	Vasodilation, BP down, HR down
Guanethidine	Inhibits norepinephrine release	Vasodilation, BP down, HR down
Clonidine	Central α_2 agonist	Vasodilation, BP down, HR down
Guanabenz	Central α_2 agonist	Vasodilation, BP down, HR down
Methyldopa	Metabolite is α_2 agonist	Vasodilation, BP down, **HR same**

Antihypertensives

*Think "**A, B, C, D**" for the four major classes of antihypertensives—ACE inhibitors, β blockers, calcium channel blockers, and diuretics.*

A Angiotensin Converting Enzyme (ACE) Inhibitors

- Common ACE inhibitors are capto**pril,** enala**pril,** and lisino**pril.**
- ACE raises blood pressure by two mechanisms, and ACE inhibitors therefore lower blood pressure by inhibiting these two actions.
  - (1) ACE converts angiotensin I to angiotensin II.
    - ○ Angiotensin II is the most potent known vasoconstrictor. It also stimulates thirst, aldosterone production, and vasopressin release, all of which increase blood pressure.
    - ○ ACE inhibitors reduce angiotensin II levels, resulting in **vasodilation,** volume depletion, and lower blood pressure.
  - (2) ACE degrades bradykinin, a potent arteriole dilator and mediator of pain ("bradypainin"). ACE inhibitors increase bradykinin levels and thereby decrease blood pressure. This is counterintuitive because pain causes increased blood pressure.
- Side effects include **cough** (common) and fatal angioedema (rare).

B Beta-Adrenergic Receptor Blockers

- Common β blockers include propranolol and metoprolol.
- β blockers decrease heart rate and cardiac output.
- β blockers cause bronchoconstriction. Do not use them in patients with asthma or chronic obstructive pulmonary disease (COPD).

C Calcium Channel Blockers

- Examples include nifedipine, diltiazem, and verapamil.
- Calcium channel blockers reduce calcium influx into vascular smooth muscle, inhibiting contraction and resulting in **vasodilation.** Decreased calcium influx also slows the conduction system of the heart.
- Side effects include **constipation** due to inhibition of smooth muscle contraction in the gut.

D Diuretics

- **All diuretics cause volume depletion by increasing excretion of Na1 and water.**
- Loop diuretics are notorious for causing K^+ depletion and **hypokalemia.**
- Thiazide diuretics can also cause hypokalemia.
- K^+-sparing diuretics can cause <u>**hyper**kalemia</u> because they inhibit K^+ secretion.

- α Adrenergic blockers cause relaxation of vascular smooth muscle by blockade of α_1 receptors.
- Direct-acting vasodilators include hydralazine (used to treat preeclampsia), minoxidil (also used for male pattern baldness), and nitroprusside (converted to nitric oxide and metabolized to cyanide).

Cholinergic Drugs

- The neurotransmitter of sympathetic and parasympathetic synapses is acetylcholine. The only relevant exceptions are sympathetic synapses, which use norepinephrine.
- There are two general classes of cholinergic receptors, nicotinic and muscarinic. Drugs affecting these receptors are presented in the following two diagrams.

Cholinergic Drugs: Nicotinic

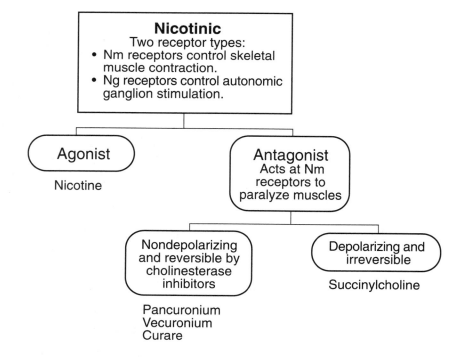

Cholinergic Drugs: Muscarinic

Muscarinic
Receptor types are not clinically important.

Agonist

Acetylcholine
Carbachol
Pilocarpine
Bethanechol ⌐ Used to treat non-obstructive urinary retention

Cholinesterase Inhibitor:
Inhibits the breakdown of acetylcholine

Organophosphates —In insecticides; antidote is atropine or pralidoxime

Edrophonium ——Myasthenia gravis diagnosis; very short acting

Pyridostigmine ——Myasthenia gravis treatment

All clinical cholinergic agonists and cholinesterase inhibitors have all of the muscarinic effects listed below.

Organ	Muscarinic Receptor Effect
Heart	Slows rate and decreases conduction velocity and atrial contractility
Lungs	Causes bronchoconstriction and increases secretions
Gut	Increases motility (diarrhea); secretes pepsin and acid
Bladder	Causes urination (contracts detrusor and relaxes sphincter)
Glands	Increases secretion
Penis	Causes erection
Eye	Constricts pupil (*Mnemonic: Miosis has two little "eyes"*); mediates accommodation

Elmer Fudd's mnemonic for effects of muscarinic receptors: "People become wet and wheezing with a swow heartbeat, wittle pupils, and an ewection." And wemember, these people are weally wet. They drool, sweat, tear, pee, poop, and secrete into their bronchi, stomachs, and other pwaces.

Avoid muscarinic drugs in cases of asthma, peptic ulcer disease, and mechanical bladder obstruction because they cause bronchoconstriction, acid secretion, and bladder contraction.

Antagonist

Atropine —— Used to treat organophosphate poisoning
Ipratroprium ⌐ Reduces bronchial secretions in COPD patients
Scopolamine ⌐ Prevents motion sickness

Muscarinic antagonists cause the opposite of the muscarinic agonist effects listed above. The patient experiences tachycardia, bronchodilation, constipation, urinary retention, **dry eyes and mouth**, decreased sweating, and mydriasis.

Other Cardiovascular Drugs

Nitrates
- Use nitrates, β-blockers, and calcium channel blockers to treat angina.
- Nitroglycerin is short-acting. Isosorbide dinitrate is long-acting.
- Tolerance to nitrates occurs rapidly, so **patches and paste must be removed overnight.**

Anticoagulants and Antithrombotic Agents

Drug	Mechanism	Relevant Side Effects
Warfarin	Blocks vitamin K*	Bleeding
Heparin	Activates antithrombin III	Bleeding
Aspirin	**Kills cyclooxygenase**	GI ulcers, asthma
Ticlopidine	Blocks platelet binding to fibrinogen	Neutropenia

*Clotting factors killed by warfarin (vitamin K dependent factors): Prothrombin (II), VII, IX, and X as well as protein C and protein S.
GI = gastrointestinal.

Thrombolytic Agents
- Thrombolytic agents enhance conversion of plasminogen to plasmin. Plasmin in turn dissolves clots by digesting fibrin and fibrinogen.
- **Bleeding** is the important side effect.
- Thrombolytics include tissue plasminogen activator, streptokinase, and urokinase.

Antiarrhythmic Agents
- This complicated group of drugs is relatively low yield.
- **Quinidine prolongs the PR interval and causes GI upset, cinchonism (headache and tinnitus), and visual disturbances.**

Cardiac Glycosides
- Digoxin and digitoxin treat heart failure and some arrhythmias.
- **Digoxin and digitoxin inhibit Na^+/K^+-ATPase.** This causes the Na^+ in heart muscle cells to rise. The elevated Na^+ drives Ca^{2+} into the cell through the Na^+/Ca^{2+} exchanger, **indirectly increasing intracellular Ca^{2+}.** Elevated intracellular Ca^{2+} strengthens heart contractions, promoting increased cardiac output.
- Digoxin and digitoxin can cause **visual disturbances, arrhythmias, and GI upset.**
- Digoxin prolongs the PR interval and shortens the QT interval on electrocardiogram (ECG).
- Factors predisposing to digoxin and digitoxin toxicity include hypokalemia (secondary to diuretics or steroids), hypercalcemia, quinidine, and amiodarone.

Lipid Lowering Agents

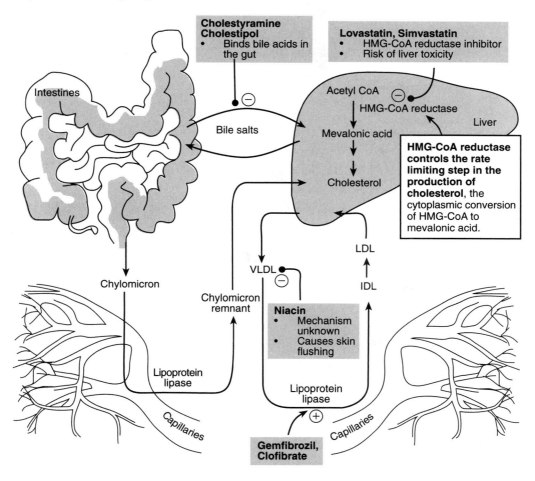

Cholestyramine Cholestipol
- Binds bile acids in the gut

Lovastatin, Simvastatin
- HMG-CoA reductase inhibitor
- Risk of liver toxicity

Intestines

Bile salts

Acetyl CoA
HMG-CoA reductase
Mevalonic acid
Cholesterol
Liver

HMG-CoA reductase controls the rate limiting step in the production of cholesterol, the cytoplasmic conversion of HMG-CoA to mevalonic acid.

LDL

VLDL

IDL

Chylomicron

Chylomicron remnant

Niacin
- Mechanism unknown
- Causes skin flushing

Lipoprotein lipase

Lipoprotein lipase

Capillaries

Capillaries

Gemfibrozil, Clofibrate

Psychoactive Drugs

Side effects of neuroleptics, tricyclic antidepressants (TCAs), and monoamine oxidase inhibitors (MAOIs) are important.

Antipsychotics
- Antipsychotics are used to treat schizophrenia and hallucinations.
- Almost all antipsychotics **block dopamine D_2 receptors.**
- Antipsychotics can be divided into two groups: low potency and high potency.
  - *(1)* **Low potency** antipsychotics: **chlorpromazine** and thioridazine
    - These are "dirty" drugs with **many immediate side effects,** including antihistaminergic (sedation, weight gain), anti-adrenergic (anti-α_2 with hypotension and reflex tachycardia), and anticholinergic effects.

(2) **High potency** antipsychotics: **haloperidol** and thiothixene
- These are more specific for dopamine receptors (D_2) and have few immediate side effects. However, there is an increased long-term risk for **parkinsonism,** tardive dyskinesia (involuntary writhing facial and trunk movements), and the deadly neuroleptic malignant syndrome.
- New high potency drugs (**clozapine**) are thought to work on D_1 or serotonin receptors. These drugs have few immediate or long-term side effects but may cause deadly **agranulocytosis** (rare). Clozapine is the only treatment for negative symptoms of schizophrenia (e.g., apathy).

- Antipsychotics may cause galactorrhea and hyperprolactinemia by blocking dopamine receptors in the pituitary.

Lithium
- Lithium is used most often for bipolar disorder (manic-depression).
- Important side effects include **hypothyroidism,** tremor, and arrhythmias.

Psychomotor Stimulants

Drug	Mechanism	Notes
Methylphenidate	Releases norepinephrine, dopamine	For attention deficit disorder
d-Amphetamine	Releases norepinephrine, dopamine	

Antidepressants
- Specific names of antidepressants are low yield except for drugs with special side effects.
- TCAs
  - TCAs block reuptake of norepinephrine, dopamine, and serotonin into neurons.
  - Side effects of TCAs include sedation, anticholinergic effects, and hypotension (from blockage of α_2 adrenergic receptors).
  - Overdose of TCAs can cause deadly cardiac arrhythmias due to increased catecholamines.
- Selective serotonin reuptake inhibitors (SSRIs)
  - SSRIs are more selective for serotonin, and have fewer anticholinergic effects and less cardiac toxicity.
- MAOIs
  - MAOIs block metabolism of norepinephrine, dopamine, and serotonin.

- Because of the inhibition of catecholamine degradation, MAOIs predispose patients to **hypertensive crises** with sympathomimetics. Cold remedies and the **tyramine** in cheese and beer can be sufficient to precipitate a crisis.
- MAOIs are deadly when used with TCAs, SSRIs, or meperidine.
- MAOIs can treat phobias.

Group	*Examples*	*Notes*
SSRI	Fluoxetine	Trade name: Prozac
	Paroxetine	
	Sertraline	
TCA	Clomipramine	For **obsessive-compulsive disorder**
	Amoxapine	Can cause neuroleptic malignant syndrome
	Nortriptyline	
	Amitriptyline	Highly sedating
	Doxepin	Highly sedating
	Imipramine	Arrhythmias; enuresis (bed wetting)
	Desipramine	Sudden death in children
MAOI	Tranylcypromine	**Hypertensive cheese crisis**
	Selegiline	MAO-B only; much safer; anti-Parkinson's
Other	Trazodone	Can cause priapism

Other Central Nervous System Drugs

Opioids

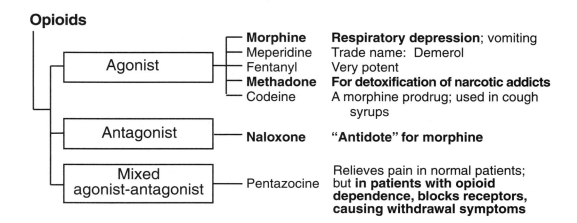

Opioids			
Agonist	—	**Morphine**	**Respiratory depression**; vomiting
	—	Meperidine	Trade name: Demerol
	—	Fentanyl	Very potent
	—	**Methadone**	**For detoxification of narcotic addicts**
	—	Codeine	A morphine prodrug; used in cough syrups
Antagonist	—	**Naloxone**	**"Antidote" for morphine**
Mixed agonist-antagonist	—	Pentazocine	Relieves pain in normal patients; but **in patients with opioid dependence, blocks receptors, causing withdrawal symptoms**

Barbiturates and Benzodiazepines

- These drugs are sedatives, antianxiety agents, and anticonvulsants.
- They bind receptors adjacent to (γ-aminobutyric acid (GABA) receptors in neurons, thus potentiating chloride flux into the cell (hyperpolarizes neurons).
- **Barbiturate *withdrawal* can be fatal.**
- **Barbiturate overdose can be fatal** because of CNS and respiratory depression.
- Barbiturates induce the cytochrome P-450 system, thereby affecting the metabolism of other drugs.
- All relevant barbiturates end in **-tal.**
    ○ Phenobarbi**tal** is the classic barbiturate.
- Most relevant benzodiazepines end in **-pam** or **-lam.**
    ○ Diaze**pam** is commonly used for muscle relaxation.

Anticonvulsants

Treatment of Choice	Seizure Type	Seizure Symptoms or Signs
Ethosuximide	**Absence**	**Staring spells, 3/sec spike and wave on EEG**
Phenytoin, carbamazepine	Focal	Unconscious or focal neurologic symptom
Phenytoin, carbamazepine	Tonic–clonic	Unconscious with tonic–clonic activity
Phenobarbital	Febrile	Young children
Phenytoin, diazepam	Status epilepticus	A rapid succession of seizures

EEG = electroencephalogram.

- **Phenytoin and carbamazepine** stabilize neuronal membranes, thereby decreasing Na^+ and K^+ currents during action potentials. Side effects include ataxia and hepatotoxicity.
- Phenytoin may cause gingival hyperplasia.
- Carbamazepine may cause aplastic anemia.
- Valproic acid may cause fatal hepatotoxicity.

General Anesthetics

- The mechanisms of general anesthetics are not known.

Drug	Type	Notes
Halothane	Inhaled	**Halothane hepatotoxicity**
Isoflurane	Inhaled	
Nitrous oxide	Inhaled	Insufficient alone
Thiopental	Injected	**Short half-life due to fat redistribution,** barbiturate

Drug	Mechanism
Levodopa	Metabolized to dopamine in CNS and periphery
Carbidopa	Increases levodopa availability by **inhibiting peripheral dopamine carboxylase;** given with levodopa
Selegiline	MAO-B inhibitor; inhibits dopamine breakdown
Bromocriptine	Powerful dopamine D_2 agonist

Antiemetics

Drug	Mechanism	Notes
Ondansetron	**Serotonin 5-HT$_3$ antagonist**	Used with chemotherapy
Prochlorperazine	Dopamine D_2 antagonist	
Promethazine	Dopamine D_2 antagonist	Also an H_1 antagonist
Metoclopramide	Dopamine D_2 antagonist	
Scopolamine	Central anticholinergic	

Chemotherapy and Immunosuppressants

- Toxicity and mechanism of action are emphasized.
- With few exceptions, one does *not* need to know what drug is used for which cancer.
- Drugs that inhibit DNA or RNA synthesis or mitosis generally kill *any* proliferating cells, leading to **bone marrow suppression, severe GI problems, and alopecia** (baldness).

Immunosuppressants

Drug	Mechanism	Notes
Cyclosporine	**Inhibits T cells by reducing IL-2**	Nephrotoxicity
Azathioprine	Metabolite inhibits purine synthesis	Cells cannot make DNA or RNA
Glucocorticoids	Multiple mechanisms	Cushing's syndrome

IL = interleukin.

Chemotherapy Agents: Mechanisms

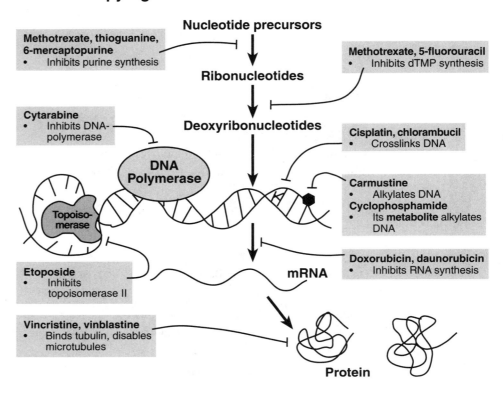

Nucleotide precursors

Methotrexate, thioguanine, 6-mercaptopurine
- Inhibits purine synthesis

Methotrexate, 5-fluorouracil
- Inhibits dTMP synthesis

Ribonucleotides

Cytarabine
- Inhibits DNA-polymerase

Deoxyribonucleotides

Cisplatin, chlorambucil
- Crosslinks DNA

DNA Polymerase

Topoiso-merase

Carmustine
- Alkylates DNA

Cyclophosphamide
- Its **metabolite** alkylates DNA

Doxorubicin, daunorubicin
- Inhibits RNA synthesis

Etoposide
- Inhibits topoisomerase II

mRNA

Vincristine, vinblastine
- Binds tubulin, disables microtubules

Protein

Hormonal Chemotherapy

Drug	*Mechanism*	*Use*
Tamoxifen	**Estrogen receptor antagonist**	Breast cancer
Leuprolide	**GnRH analog** *	Advanced prostate cancer

*When given continuously, leuprolide **decreases** gonadotropin release by desensitizing gonadotropin-releasing hormone (GnRH) receptors in the pituitary.

Special
- **Retinoic acid** causes malignant stem cells to **mature and differentiate,** so they drop out of the cell cycle and stop proliferating.

Chemotherapy Agents and Side Effects
- Several drug-specific side effects are often tested.

Drug	*Side Effects*
Bleomycin	**Pulmonary fibrosis**
Doxorubicin*	**Cardiomyopathy**

continued

Drug	Side Effects
Daunorubicin*	**Cardiomyopathy**
Cyclophosphamide	**Hemorrhagic cystitis,** prevented with *N*-acetylcysteine or MESNA
Methotrexate	Myelosuppression, stomatitis, prevented with leucovorin
Vincristine	Peripheral neuropathy, **no myelosuppression**
5-Fluorouracil	Cerebellar toxicity, myelosuppression
Cisplatin	Nephrotoxicity, ototoxicity

Mnemonic: "Heart rub." Cardiomyopathy is caused by chemotherapeutic drugs with "rub" in the name.

Drugs For Bronchial Disease

- **Albuterol is the drug of choice for most asthma.**
- **Cromolyn prevents mast cell degranulation.** It is used for asthma prophylaxis only.
- Theophylline and aminophylline inhibit phosphodiesterase, thus increasing cyclic adenosine monophosphate (cAMP). Furthermore, they inhibit adenosine receptors. These actions lead to bronchodilation. They have a narrow therapeutic index.
- **Ipratropium decreases bronchial secretions.**
- Epinephrine is used in emergencies for severe bronchoconstriction.
- Glucocorticoids, such as beclomethasone and prednisone, are commonly used to decrease inflammation.

Peptic Ulcer Drugs

Drug	Mechanism	Relevant Side Effects
Cimetidine	**H_2 antagonist**	**Inhibits P-450 system**
Ranitidine	H_2 antagonist	Few side effects
Omeprazole	Inhibits H^+/K^+-ATPase	Few side effects
Antacids	Neutralizes acid	**Constipation** (or diarrhea, with Mg^{2+} antacids); inhibits absorption of tetracycline, ciprofloxacin ketoconazole, isoniazid, and aspirin
Bismuth salicylate	Kills *Helicobacter pylori*	Black stools; salicylism
Sucralfate	Coats the stomach mucosa	Few side effects; cannot be used with antacids

Gout Drugs

Drug	Mechanism	Notes
Allopurinol	**Inhibits xanthine oxidase**	Lowers uric acid; for gout prophylaxis Initial doses may precipitate an acute attack
Colchicine	Breaks down microtubules thus inhibiting inflammatory cell chemotaxis into the joint	For acute attacks of gout

Antipyretics

- Aspirin, ibuprofen, and indomethacin are examples of nonsteroidal anti-inflammatory drugs (NSAIDs).
- **All NSAIDs inhibit cyclooxygenase,** a critical enzyme in the formation of prostaglandins from arachidonic acid.
- Aspirin toxicity (salicylism) initially causes respiratory stimulation, then respiratory depression and failure. Other symptoms include tinnitus, vomiting, and confusion. Chronic overdose causes respiratory alkalosis with metabolic acidosis.
- Indomethacin is used to close patent ductus arteriosus in newborns.

Toxicology

tylenol

Drug	Syndrome	Antidote
Acetaminophen	**Hepatic necrosis**	**N-acetylcysteine**
Opioids	Respiratory depression	**Naloxone**
Organophosphates	Muscarinic agonist effects	Atropine, pralidoxime
Heparin	Bleeding	Protamine
Warfarin	Bleeding	Vitamin K, fresh frozen plasma
Atropine	Anticholinergic effects	Physostigmine
Methanol	Blindness	Ethanol
Lead	Encephalopathy, anemia	EDTA, dimercaprol
TCAs	Cardiac arrhythmia	Sodium bicarbonate
Digitalis	Cardiac arrhythmia	Lidocaine, anti-digitalis Fab fragments

continued

Drug	Syndrome	Antidote
Succinylcholine	Malignant hyperthermia	Dantrolene (inhibits Ca^{2+} release from sarcoplasmic reticulum, thus preventing muscle contraction and heat generation)

EDTA = ethylenediaminetetraacetic acid.

Important Drug–Drug Interactions and Interferences

Drugs	Interaction
MAOIs—levodopa	Hypertensive crisis due to increased catecholamines
MAOIs—TCAs	Hypertensive crisis (both have adrenergic effects)
TCAs—CNS depressants/ethanol	Toxic sedation
Quinidine—digitalis	Increases digitalis levels

High-Yield Side Effects

Side Effect	Drugs
Teratogen (birth defects)	Isotretinoin, retinoic acid, diethylstilbestrol, anticonvulsants, ethanol, warfarin
Aplastic anemia	Carbamazepine, chloramphenicol
Crystalluria	Methotrexate, sulfonamides
Lupus-like syndromes	Procainamide, hydralazine
Stevens-Johnson syndrome	Sulfonamides
Photosensitivity	Retinoic acid, tetracyclines, amiodarone
Venous thrombosis	Oral contraceptives

- **Isoniazid** may cause **peripheral neuritis unless taken with vitamin B_6** (pyridoxine), and may also cause **hepatitis.**

Look-Alikes

Drugs	Effects
Metaproterenol	Long-lasting β_2 agonist, bronchodilator; inhaled
Metoprolol	Cardioselective β blocker (β_1)
Clotrimazole	Topical antifungal
Cotrimoxazole	Sulfa drug/antibiotic

Biochemistry

CHAPTER 5

Christina Kahl

Coach's Tips

- Rate-limiting steps in biochemical pathways are the highest yield.
- Regulation of rate-limiting enzymes is high yield.
- Vitamin deficiencies and inherited defects that cause disease are high yield.
- DNA and RNA synthesis are moderate yield.
- Molecular biology and receptor subtypes are moderate yield.
- Molecular structures are low yield.

Amino Acids

- Amino acids with acidic side chains are aspartate and glutamate.
- Amino acids with basic side chains are histidine, lysine, and arginine.
- The two ketogenic amino acids are lysine and leucine.
- The essential amino acids are *a*rginine, *h*istidine, *m*ethionine, *t*hreonine, *t*ryptophan, *l*eucine, *p*henylalanine, *i*soleucine, *l*ysine, and *v*aline.

Mnemonic: **A H**ungry **M**ob **T**hreatened **T**o **L**ynch **P**eople **I**ngesting **L**eafy **V**egetables.

Enzyme Kinetics

- **Michaelis constant** (K_m) is the concentration of substrate that produces half of the maximal enzyme velocity (V_{max}). A **low K_m** means the enzyme has a **high affinity** for the substrate.
- **Competitive inhibitors** reversibly bind enzymes at the same site as the substrate. The presence of competitive inhibitors will increase the apparent K_m but will not change the V_{max}.
- **Noncompetitive inhibitors** bind enzymes at a different site than the substrate. Noncompetitive inhibitors decrease the V_{max} but do not change K_m.

Hemoglobin

- In hemoglobin, the iron is in the **ferrous state (Fe^{2+})**.
- Adult hemoglobin (HbA) is composed of two α and two β subunits.
- Fetal hemoglobin (HbF) is composed of two α and two **γ subunits.**

- **HbA$_{1c}$** is the glycosylated form of hemoglobin. HbA$_{1c}$ forms spontaneously in the blood in the presence of glucose. Elevated HbA$_{1c}$ levels result from chronically uncontrolled diabetes mellitus.
- In **sickle cell anemia,** the β subunit contains a glutamate to valine mutation at position 6.
- In **α-thalassemia,** synthesis of normal α subunits is decreased or absent.
- In **β-thalassemia,** synthesis of normal β subunits is decreased or absent.

Heme Synthesis and Degradation

Synthesis
- The rate-limiting enzyme in porphyrin biosynthesis is δ-aminolevulinic acid **(ALA) synthase,** which converts glycine and succinyl coenzyme A (CoA) to ALA.

Degradation
- Macrophages scavenge old heme and convert it to biliverdin and then to **bilirubin.**
- Bilirubin–albumin complexes travel in the bloodstream to the **liver,** which **conjugates** bilirubin to form **bilirubin diglucuronide.**
- The liver excretes these conjugates (bile) into the intestines where they are converted to **urobilinogen.**
- Although most of the bilirubin gets excreted, a small portion is reabsorbed and excreted by the kidney as **urobilin.**
- **Indirect bilirubin** measures **unconjugated** bilirubin, primarily the bilirubin–albumin complexes in the bloodstream. **Direct bilirubin** measures the **conjugated** form, bilirubin diglucuronide.

Collagen and Elastin

- **Collagen** is a glycoprotein composed of three peptides wrapped in a triple helix. The amino acids are repeating triplets of glycine-X-Y, where X and Y are often **hydroxylated** proline and lysine. **Vitamin C** is required for this hydroxylation, and lack of vitamin C leads to scurvy, a disease of poor collagen formation.
- Once in the extracellular matrix, **lysyl oxidase** crosslinks collagen helices to one another to form a matrix.
- Collagen type IV is present in basement membranes. Collagen type II is found in cartilage.
- **Ehlers-Danlos syndrome** is due to defective collagen synthesis and is characterized by stretchy skin and hyperflexible joints.
- **Elastin** is also rich in proline and lysine, but is not hydroxylated.

Elastin is protected from degradation by α_1-antitrypsin. **α_1-Antitrypsin deficiency** leads to emphysema and hepatitis.

Electron Transport Chain

- The electron transport chain proteins are on the inner mitochondrial membrane. The electron transport chain is made of five complexes (I, II, III, IV, and V) where adenosine triphosphate (ATP) synthetase is complex V.

- Electrons from reduced nicotinamide adenine dinucleotide (NADH) and reduced flavin adenine dinucleotide (FADH$_2$) are passed down through complexes I, II, III, and IV. This causes H$^+$ to be pumped out from inside the mitochondria, producing an H$^+$ gradient.

Electron Transport Chain

Components and their inhibitors

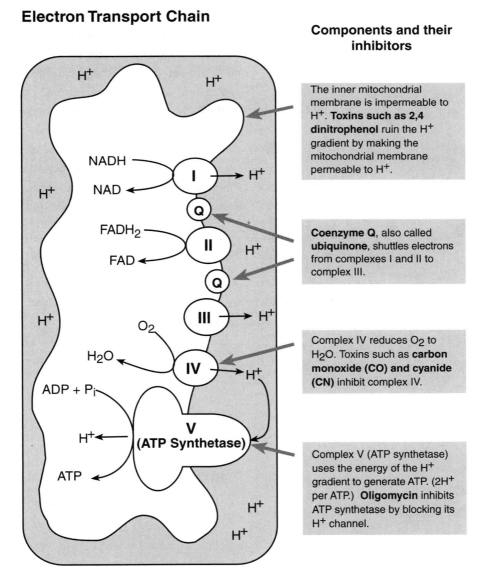

The inner mitochondrial membrane is impermeable to H$^+$. **Toxins such as 2,4 dinitrophenol** ruin the H$^+$ gradient by making the mitochondrial membrane permeable to H$^+$.

Coenzyme Q, also called **ubiquinone,** shuttles electrons from complexes I and II to complex III.

Complex IV reduces O$_2$ to H$_2$O. Toxins such as **carbon monoxide (CO) and cyanide (CN)** inhibit complex IV.

Complex V (ATP synthetase) uses the energy of the H$^+$ gradient to generate ATP. (2H$^+$ per ATP.) **Oligomycin** inhibits ATP synthetase by blocking its H$^+$ channel.

Metabolism

- When reviewing these pathways, pay attention to (1) **control points** and rate-limiting steps and (2) **cofactors.** The actions of insulin and glucagon are particularly important (see table below).

	Insulin	*Glucagon*
Secretion	β-Cells (pancreas) + Glucose, secretin − Epinephrine, somatostatin	α-Cells (pancreas) + Epinephrine, hypoglycemia − Insulin, somatostatin
Receptor	Tyrosine kinase receptor	G-protein-coupled receptor
Signal pathway	Lowers cAMP Promotes dephosphorylation	Activates AC to increase cAMP Promotes phosphorylation
Carbohydrates	Promotes glycolysis and glycogen synthesis	Promotes gluconeogenesis and glycogen degradation
Lipids	Activates lipoprotein lipase and triglyceride synthesis	Activates hormone-sensitive lipase and oxidation of fatty acids to ketone bodies
Protein	Promotes amino acid synthesis	Promotes amino acid breakdown (gluconeo-genesis)

AC = adenylate cyclase; cAMP = cyclic adenosine monophosphate.

- Tricky point: Glucagon increases insulin secretion, whereas insulin decreases glucagon secretion. Somatostatin decreases secretion of both insulin and glucagon.

Glycolysis

- Glycolysis is turned *on* in the liver by **insulin** and **glucose.**
- Glycolysis is turned *off* in the liver by **glucagon, epinephrine, intracellular citrate, and ATP.**

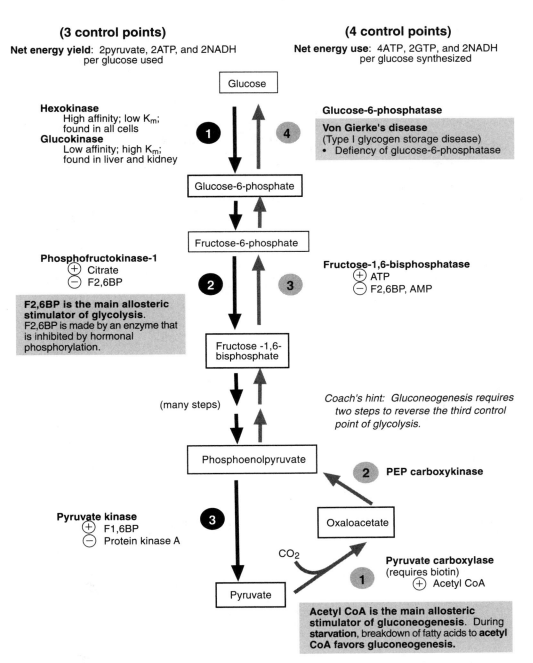

(3 control points)

Net energy yield: 2pyruvate, 2ATP, and 2NADH
per glucose used

(4 control points)

Net energy use: 4ATP, 2GTP, and 2NADH
per glucose synthesized

Glucose

Hexokinase
High affinity; low K_m;
found in all cells
Glucokinase
Low affinity; high K_m;
found in liver and kidney

Glucose-6-phosphatase

Von Gierke's disease
(Type I glycogen storage disease)
- Defiency of glucose-6-phosphatase

Glucose-6-phosphate

Fructose-6-phosphate

Phosphofructokinase-1
(+) Citrate
(−) F2,6BP

F2,6BP is the main allosteric stimulator of glycolysis.
F2,6BP is made by an enzyme that is inhibited by hormonal phosphorylation.

Fructose-1,6-bisphosphatase
(+) ATP
(−) F2,6BP, AMP

Fructose -1,6-bisphosphate

(many steps)

Coach's hint: Gluconeogenesis requires two steps to reverse the third control point of glycolysis.

Phosphoenolpyruvate

2 **PEP carboxykinase**

Pyruvate kinase
(+) F1,6BP
(−) Protein kinase A

Oxaloacetate

CO_2

Pyruvate

1

Pyruvate carboxylase
(requires biotin)
(+) Acetyl CoA

Acetyl CoA is the main allosteric stimulator of gluconeogenesis. During **starvation**, breakdown of fatty acids to **acetyl CoA favors gluconeogenesis.**

Coach's hint: Everything in the diagram above occurs in the cytoplasm except for the pyruvate carboxylase step (step 1 to 2 in the gluconeogenesis pathway), which occurs in the mitochondria.

TCA Cycle
(5 control points)

Net yield: 3NADH, 2CO$_2$, FADH$_2$, GTP, CoA
from each acetyl CoA (12 ATP per acetyl CoA)

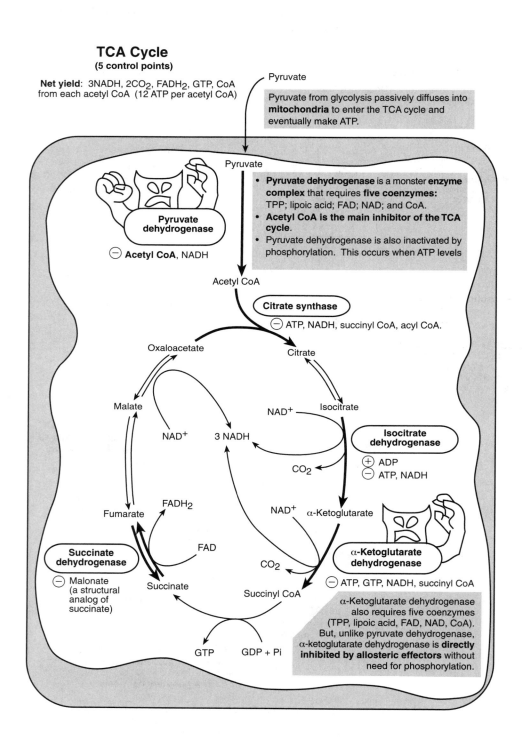

Pyruvate

Pyruvate from glycolysis passively diffuses into **mitochondria** to enter the TCA cycle and eventually make ATP.

Pyruvate

- **Pyruvate dehydrogenase** is a monster **enzyme complex** that requires **five coenzymes:** TPP; lipoic acid; FAD; NAD; and CoA.
- **Acetyl CoA is the main inhibitor of the TCA cycle**.
- Pyruvate dehydrogenase is also inactivated by phosphorylation. This occurs when ATP levels

Pyruvate dehydrogenase

⊖ **Acetyl CoA**, NADH

Acetyl CoA

Citrate synthase

⊖ ATP, NADH, succinyl CoA, acyl CoA.

Oxaloacetate

Citrate

Malate

Isocitrate

NAD$^+$

NAD$^+$

3 NADH

Isocitrate dehydrogenase

⊕ ADP
⊖ ATP, NADH

CO$_2$

Fumarate

FADH$_2$

NAD$^+$

α-Ketoglutarate

FAD

α-Ketoglutarate dehydrogenase

Succinate dehydrogenase

CO$_2$

⊖ Malonate
(a structural analog of succinate)

Succinate

Succinyl CoA

⊖ ATP, GTP, NADH, succinyl CoA

α-Ketoglutarate dehydrogenase also requires five coenzymes (TPP, lipoic acid, FAD, NAD, CoA). But, unlike pyruvate dehydrogenase, α-ketoglutarate dehydrogenase is **directly inhibited by allosteric effectors** without need for phosphorylation.

GTP

GDP + Pi

Glycogen

- Liver and muscle store glucose in the form of glycogen. Glycogen gets rapidly mobilized when glucose is needed. Extensive branching makes glycogen more soluble.

Glycogen Synthesis

- Glycogen synthesis occurs in the cytoplasm and requires ATP. Glucose-6-phosphate and insulin stimulate glycogen synthesis.
- Free glucose-6-phosphate is converted to glucose-1-phosphate, which is then converted to uridine diphosphate (UDP)-glucose.
- **Glycogen synthase** binds UDP-glucose to growing glycogen molecules via α-1,4 linkages.
- Glucosyl transferase, also called the branching enzyme, forms α-1,6 linkages in glycogen to create the branching structure.

Glycogenolysis

- Glycogen phosphorylase breaks down glycogen to glucose-1-phosphate and the debranching enzyme removes branches.
- Glycogenolysis is stimulated by epinephrine, glucagon, calcium, and AMP.
- Enzyme phosphorylation states determine if glycogenolysis is on or off. Epinephrine and glucagon stimulate adenylate cyclase to increase cAMP levels and activate protein kinase A (PKA). PKA phosphorylates glycogen synthase a (active) to form glycogen synthase b (inactive) and turn off glycogen synthesis. Furthermore, phosphorylase kinase turns on glycogenolysis by phosphorylating glycogen phosphorylase b (inactive) to form glycogen phosphorylase a (active).

Glycogen Storage Diseases

- These genetic defects result in abnormal accumulation of glycogen in specific tissues.

Disease	*Deficiency*	*Manifestations*
Von Gierke's (I)	Glucose-6-phosphatase	Hepatomegaly, fasting hypoglycemia
Pompe's (II)	Lysosomal α-glucosidase	Cardiomegaly, early death
McArdle's (V)	Muscle glycogen phosphorylase	Cramping after exercise, myoglobinuria

Hexose Monophosphate Pathway (HMP)

- The HMP pathway, also called the pentose phosphate pathway, occurs in the cytoplasm.
- The main regulated step is the irreversible oxidation of glucose-6-phosphate by **glucose-6-phosphate dehydrogenase (G6PD).** This step requires oxidized nicotinamide adenine dinucleotide phosphate ($NADP^+$) as a coenzyme and is inhibited by high levels of reduced nicotinamide adenine dinucleotide phosphate (NADPH).
- The HMP pathway generates NADPH and ribose phosphate.
- NADPH is necessary for detoxification of dangerous free radical species, reductive biosynthesis of fatty acids and sterols, and reactions in the liver P-450 system.
- Patients with G6PD deficiency are at risk for hemolytic anemia because red blood cells depend on the HMP pathway to generate NADPH. G6PD deficiency is X-linked recessive and commonly occurs in African-Americans. Antibiotics, antimalarials, antipyretics, and infection trigger hemolysis.
- The HMP pathway also generates **ribose-5-phosphate,** a molecule used by transketolases and transaldolases to synthesize nucleotides and glycolysis intermediates.

Coach's hint: *Be aware, an alternate pathway to generate NADPH is via NADPH-dependent malate dehydrogenase.*

Fatty Acid Metabolism

Fatty Acid Synthesis   versus   Fatty Acid Breakdown

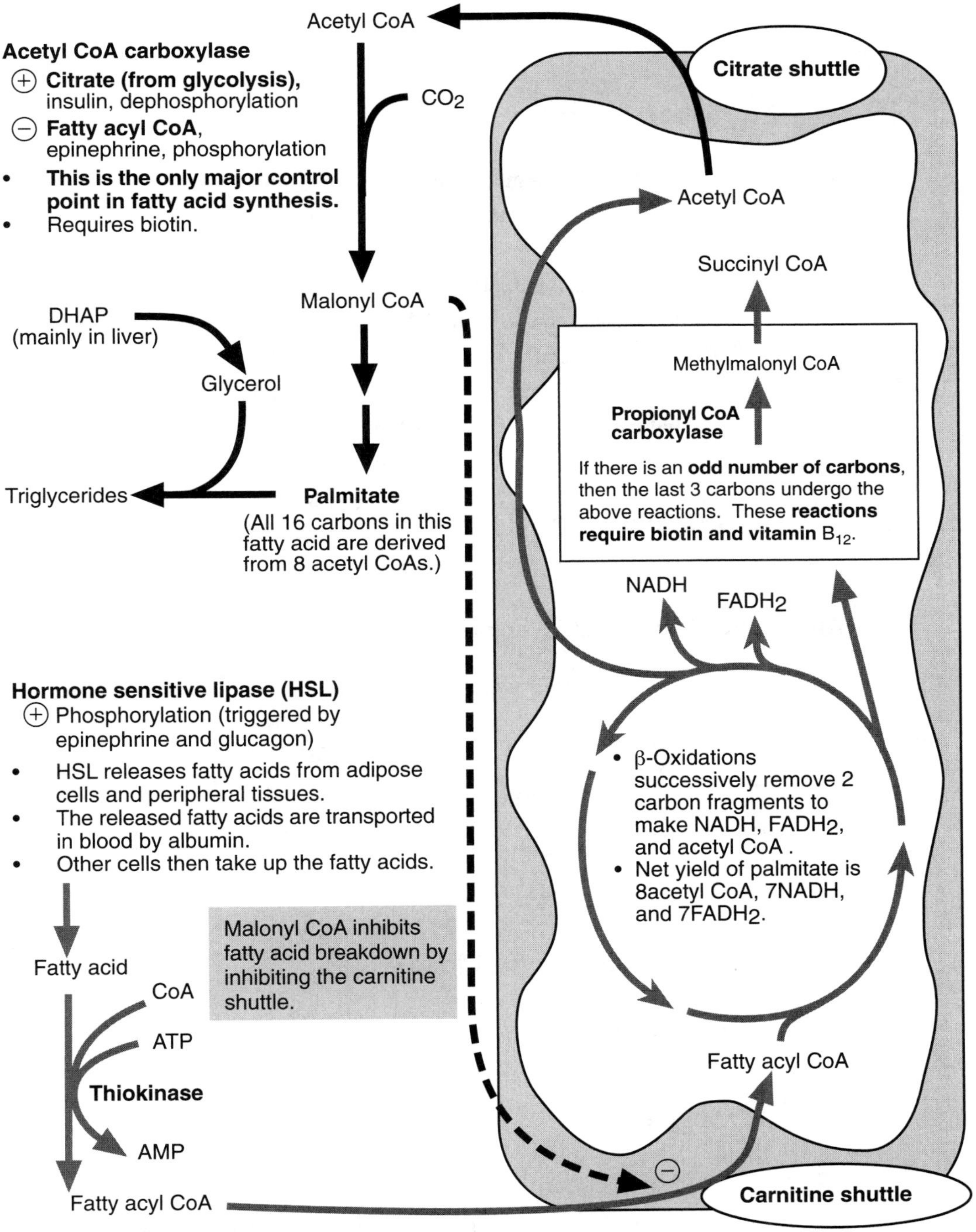

Acetyl CoA

Acetyl CoA carboxylase

$\oplus$ **Citrate (from glycolysis),** insulin, dephosphorylation

$\ominus$ **Fatty acyl CoA,** epinephrine, phosphorylation

- **This is the only major control point in fatty acid synthesis.**
- Requires biotin.

CO_2

DHAP (mainly in liver)

Glycerol

Malonyl CoA

Triglycerides

Palmitate
(All 16 carbons in this fatty acid are derived from 8 acetyl CoAs.)

Citrate shuttle

Acetyl CoA

Succinyl CoA

Methylmalonyl CoA

Propionyl CoA carboxylase

If there is an **odd number of carbons**, then the last 3 carbons undergo the above reactions. These **reactions require biotin and vitamin B_{12}.**

NADH $FADH_2$

Hormone sensitive lipase (HSL)

$\oplus$ Phosphorylation (triggered by epinephrine and glucagon)

- HSL releases fatty acids from adipose cells and peripheral tissues.
- The released fatty acids are transported in blood by albumin.
- Other cells then take up the fatty acids.

Fatty acid

CoA

ATP

Thiokinase

AMP

Fatty acyl CoA

Malonyl CoA inhibits fatty acid breakdown by inhibiting the carnitine shuttle.

- β-Oxidations successively remove 2 carbon fragments to make NADH, $FADH_2$, and acetyl CoA.
- Net yield of palmitate is 8acetyl CoA, 7NADH, and $7FADH_2$.

Fatty acyl CoA

$\ominus$

Carnitine shuttle

Ethanol Metabolism

- Alcohol dehydrogenase metabolizes ethanol to acetaldehyde by zero-order kinetics. This reaction consumes oxidized NAD (NAD^+) and increases the NADH to NAD^+ ratio. In turn, high NADH inhibits gluconeogenesis, resulting in hypoglycemia.

Ketone Bodies

- **Acetyl CoA cannot undergo gluconeogenesis,** and thus, fat cannot be converted to glucose. In the liver, acetyl CoA is converted to ketone bodies via β-hydroxy-β-methylglutaryl coenzyme A (HMG CoA) synthase and HMG CoA lyase to generate **acetoacetate.** Acetoacetate is converted to **β-hydroxybutyrate** (the major ketone body) or acetate.
- The production of ketone bodies occurs during **starvation** and **diabetic ketoacidosis.**

Deamination

Amino acid Deamination and Amination

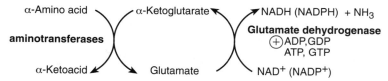

The arrows indicate pathways for amino acid degradation.
These reacions occur in reverse for amino acid synthesis.

Mucopolysaccharidoses

- These genetic defects result in incomplete degradation of glycosaminoglycans.

Disease	Deficiency	Notes
Hurler's syndrome	α-L-Iduronidase	Corneal clouding, mental retardation
Hunter's syndrome	Iduronate sulfatase	X-linked, mental retardation, deformity

Sphingolipidoses

- These genetic defects result in the accumulation of sphingolipids in certain tissues.

Disease	Deficiency	Notes
Tay-Sach's	β-Hexosaminidase A ($\uparrow$ gangliosides)	Autosomal recessive, Ashkenazic Jews, mental retardation, cherry macula
Gaucher's	β-Glucosidase ($\uparrow$ glucocerebrosides)	Autosomal recessive, hepatosplenomegaly, osteoporosis
Fabry's	α-Galactosidase ($\uparrow$ globosides)	X-linked, kidney and heart failure, rash
Niemann-Pick	Sphingomyelinase ($\uparrow$ sphingomyelin)	Autosomal recessive, hepatosplenomegaly, early death

Amino Acid Disorders

Disease	Deficiency	Notes
Phenylketonuria (PKU)	Phenylalanine hydroxylase	Mental retardation, hypopigmentation, treat with $\downarrow$ phe and $\uparrow$ try
Maple syrup urine disease	Branched-chain dehydrogenase	CNS defects, sweet odor, early death
Homocystinuria	Cystathione synthetase	Mental retardation, lens dislocation
Dislocation alkaptonuria	Homogentisate oxidase	Dark urine, benign

CNS = central nervous system; phe = phenylalanine; try = tryptophan.

Nucleotides

- **Purine** nucleotides (**A, G**) have two rings and **pyrimidine** nucleotides (**C, T, U**) have one ring. Thymidine is only in DNA and uracil is only in RNA.

Mnemonic: *Remember the alphabet—purine comes before pyrimidine. Likewise, A comes before C, and G comes before T.*

- G-C pairing has 3 H bonds and A-T (or A-U) has 2 H bonds.

Disorders of Purine Degradation and Salvage

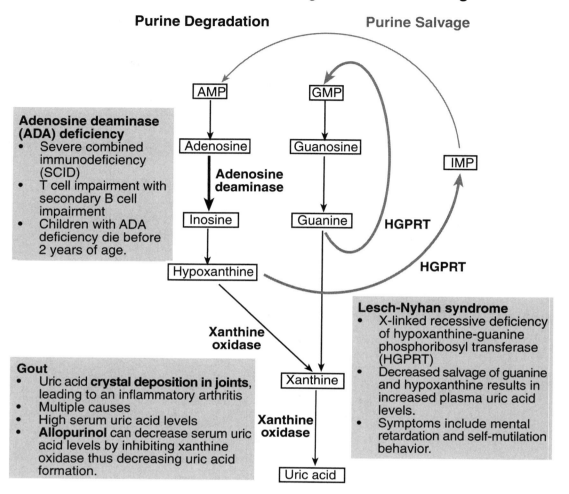

Purine Degradation

Purine Salvage

Adenosine deaminase (ADA) deficiency
- Severe combined immunodeficiency (SCID)
- T cell impairment with secondary B cell impairment
- Children with ADA deficiency die before 2 years of age.

AMP → Adenosine

Adenosine deaminase

Adenosine → Inosine → Hypoxanthine

GMP → Guanosine → Guanine

IMP

HGPRT

HGPRT

Gout
- Uric acid **crystal deposition in joints**, leading to an inflammatory arthritis
- Multiple causes
- High serum uric acid levels
- **Allopurinol** can decrease serum uric acid levels by inhibiting xanthine oxidase thus decreasing uric acid formation.

Xanthine oxidase

Xanthine

Xanthine oxidase

Uric acid

Lesch-Nyhan syndrome
- X-linked recessive deficiency of hypoxanthine-guanine phosphoribosyl transferase (HGPRT)
- Decreased salvage of guanine and hypoxanthine results in increased plasma uric acid levels.
- Symptoms include mental retardation and self-mutilation behavior.

DNA Replication

Mutations
- **Missense** mutations result in a single amino acid change.
- **Nonsense** mutations result in a premature stop codon.
- **Frameshift** mutations result in misreading of all downstream nucleotides.

RNA

- **Ribosomal RNA (rRNA)** is the most abundant form of RNA (80%) and is synthesized by **RNA polymerase I.** It associates with proteins to form **ribosomes,** the site of protein synthesis.

DNA Replication

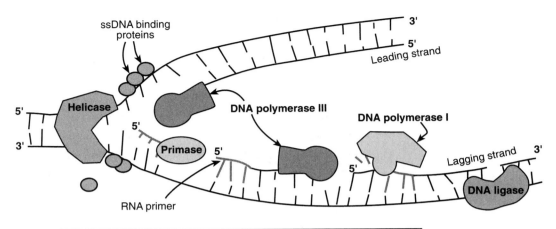

Prokaryotic enzyme	Eukaryotic equivalent	Function
Primase	pol α	Synthesizes RNA primer
DNA polymerase III	pol δ	Elongates leading strand
DNA polymerase III	pol ε	Elongates lagging strand
DNA polymerase I	pol β	5'-3' RNA exonuclease (removes RNA primer and fills the gap with DNA)

- **Messenger RNA (mRNA)** is the most heterogeneous form of RNA and is synthesized by **RNA polymerase II.**
- **Promoters** (TATA and CAAT boxes) are short DNA sequences upstream of a gene and are necessary to initiate transcription. RNA polymerase II and transcription factors bind these sequences.
- **Enhancers** are also short DNA sequences that bind transcription factors. They may be upstream, downstream, or within a gene and help regulate the transcription of the gene.
- After synthesis, mRNA undergoes three modifications. **A 7-methyl-guanosine cap** is added to the 5′ end to increase stability. A **poly-A tail** is added to the 3′ end. **Introns,** the noncoding regions, are spliced out. Differential splicing may give different protein products from a single gene. (**Exons** are the coding sequences.)

Mnemonic: ***E****xons are* ***E****xpressed.*

- **Transfer RNA (tRNA)** is the smallest RNA and is synthesized by **RNA polymerase III.** Transfer RNA has a cloverleaf structure and binds a single, specific amino acid.

Protein Synthesis

- **Aminoacyl-tRNA synthetase** covalently attaches the appropriate amino acid to the 3′ end of the tRNA to form aminoacyl-tRNA. This reaction is called **"tRNA charging"** and requires ATP.

Coach's Hint: *Ribosomes are composed of two sites. The **A site** accepts the incoming **a**minoacyl-tRNA and the **P site** binds the growing **p**eptidyl-tRNA.*

- **Initiation** begins with the assembly of two ribosomal subunits, mRNA, the first aminoacyl-tRNA, guanosine triphosphate (GTP) and several initiation factors. The first codon is always **AUG,** which specifies methionine or N-formylated methionine (f-met) in prokaryotes.

- **Elongation** continues as the mRNA is read 5′ to 3′, and amino acids are added to the carboxyl terminus of the polypeptide.

- **Termination** and release of the polypeptide occurs when a stop codon is read.

- **ATP** is required for **tRNA charging. GTP** is required for binding of the **aminoacyl-tRNA to the A site** and for **translocation.**

- After synthesis, proteins may undergo a number of post-translation modifications including cleavage, phosphorylation, glycosylation, hydroxylation, and lipid modification.

Post-Transcriptional Modification of Eukaryotic mRNA
None of these modifications occur in prokaryotes

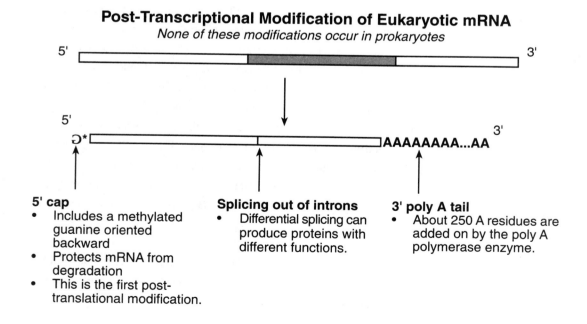

5′ cap
- Includes a methylated guanine oriented backward
- Protects mRNA from degradation
- This is the first post-translational modification.

Splicing out of introns
- Differential splicing can produce proteins with different functions.

3′ poly A tail
- About 250 A residues are added on by the poly A polymerase enzyme.

Nutrition

- The **fat-soluble vitamins** are **A, D, E, and K.** The rest are water-soluble.
- The **antioxidants** include vitamin C, vitamin E, and β-carotenes. They chemically inactivate oxygen radicals.
- **Kwashiorkor** is a defiance in **protein** intake, whereas **marasmus** is a defiance in total **caloric** intake.

Vitamin	*Biochemistry*	*Deficiency*
Thiamine (B$_1$)	TPP decarboxylations (TCA), transketolases	Beri-beri, Wernicke-Korsakoff
Riboflavin (B$_2$)	FMN, FAD oxidations and reductions	Dermatitis, cheilosis
Pyridoxine (B$_6$)	Pyridoxal phosphate transaminations, deaminations	Inducible by INH
Cobalamin (B$_{12}$)	Methionine synthesis, odd chain FA degradation	Megaloblastic anemia, neuropathy
Niacin	NAD$^+$, NADP$^+$ oxidations and reductions	Pellagra (dermatitis, dementia, diarrhea)
Biotin	Carboxylations	
Folic acid	One-carbon metabolism, nucleotide biosynthesis	Megaloblastic anemia, neural tube birth defects
Vitamin C	Hydroxylation of proline and lysine	Scurvy
Vitamin A	Part of rhodopsin, growth and reproduction	Night blindness, dry skin; EXCESS is teratogenic
Vitamin D	1,25 diOHD$_3$, intestinal absorption Ca^{2+}	Rickets, osteomalacia, renal osteodystrophy
Vitamin K	Carboxylation of glutamate, synthesis of II, VII, IX, X	Bleeding disorders
Vitamin E	Antioxidant	

diOHD$_3$ = 1,25 diOHD$_3$ = 1,25 dihydroxy vitamin D$_3$; FA = fatty acid; FMN = flavin mononucleotide; INH = isoniazid; TPP = thiamine pyrophosphate.

Signal Transduction

Receptor	Receptor class	Actions
Nicotinic acetylcholine; GABA	Ligand-gated ion channels	Changes membrane potential or ion concentrations
Insulin; Growth factors (e.g. PDGF)	Tyrosine kinases	Phosphorylation of proteins
TGF-β	Serine kinase	Phosphorylation of proteins
β₂-Adrenergic **Glucagon** **Epinephrine**	G-protein coupled	Activates AC, ↑cAMP, and activates PKA
α₁-Adrenergic	G-protein coupled	Inhibits AC and ↓ cAMP
α₁-Adrenergic Angiotensin II	G-protein coupled ADH and diacylglycerol	Activates PLC to give IP₃ IP₃ acts to ↑Ca²⁺, diacylglycerol activates PKC
Steroids Vitamin D Retinoic acid Thyroxine	Intracellular receptors	Activates gene transcription

AC = adenylate cyclase; ADH = antidiuretic hormone; GABA = γ-aminobutyric acid; IP₃ ✕ inositol 1,4,5-triphosphate; PDGF = platelet-derived growth factor; PKA = protein kinase A; PKC = protein kinase C; PLC = phospholipase C; TGF = Transforming Growth Factor B.

Coach's Hint: *Nitric oxide (or EDRF) diffuses across cellular membranes to activate a cytosolic guanylate cyclase (GC), resulting in a cyclic guanosine monophosphate (cGMP) increase and protein kinase G (PKG) activation. Nitric oxide vasodilates, relaxes smooth muscle, and inhibits platelet aggregation.*

Molecular Biology

Restriction enzymes

- **Restriction enzymes** recognize short, palindromic DNA sequences and cleave DNA into restriction fragments with "sticky" (cohesive) or blunt ends.

Coach's Hint: *Restriction enzymes were originally isolated from bacteria. Their function is to defend bacteria from invading viruses by cleaving foreign DNA.*

• A **vector** is capable of autonomous replication, carries an antibiotic resistance gene for selection, and possesses a multiple cloning site for insertion of genes. Vectors are used to generate genomic and complementary DNA (cDNA) libraries, and to express proteins.

• **PCR** rapidly and exponentially amplifies a DNA template. The reaction requires a DNA template, two oligonucleotide primers that are complementary to the template, deoxynucleoside triphosphates (dNTPs), and a heat-stable DNA polymerase such as *Taq*.

   (1) The double-stranded DNA (**dsDNA) template** is **denatured** at high temperature (94°C) to form single-stranded DNA (ssDNA).

   (2) The **primers anneal** to the ssDNA template at low temperature (30–65°C).

   (3) **DNA polymerase synthesizes new strands** of cDNA (72°C). These three steps are repeated for 30 cycles.

   • PCR is used to detect gene mutations, to detect rare nucleotide sequences (viral or bacterial DNA), and to analyze forensic samples (hair and blood).

   • RT-PCR uses an RNA template and reverse transcriptase to amplify the corresponding cDNA.

• Polymorphisms are variations in DNA sequences between some individuals. If two people have polymorphisms in a region of interest, then cleavage of their DNA by restriction enzymes will generate DNA fragments of different sizes. **RFLP** analysis refers to the comparison of such DNA fragments, looking for differences. It is used to detect gene mutations directly or through linkage analysis of polymorphisms with gene mutations.

Blots

• **Southern blots** look for the presence of a particular DNA sequence from total DNA. It is performed in the following manner:

   (1) The total **DNA** is **cleaved into fragments** using one or more restriction enzymes.

   (2) Agarose gel **electrophoresis** separates the fragments by size.

   (3) These separated fragments are **transferred** from the gel onto a sheet of **nitrocellulose filter.**

(4) The filter is **hybridized** with a **radioactive DNA probe.**

(5) The filter is exposed to film to generate an autoradiogram. This technique is used to detect gene rearrangements and deletions.

Northern blots •   **Northern blotting** follows the same principles of Southern blotting, but **mRNA** is separated by electrophoresis and **detected (hybridized) with a radiolabeled DNA probe.** It is used to detect mRNA expression in a variety of tissues or disease states.

Western blots •   In **Western blotting,** the presence of a given **protein** is sought. Cellular proteins are separated by molecular weight using SDS-PAGE (polyacrylamide system) electrophoresis. After transferring these separated proteins onto a filter, **labeled antibody** specific to the desired protein is used to detect that protein.

Physiology

CHAPTER 6

Coach's Tips

- As a general principle, the physiology underlying mechanisms of actions of major clinical drugs is important.
- Hormone production, regulation, receptors, and effects are worth learning in detail.
- The renin–angiotensin–aldosterone axis and the effects of aldosterone deficiency and excess in particular are high yield.
- Basic equations such as the Fick principle and renal clearance appear on the exam. Calculations will be simple.
- The cardiac action potential is high yield.

Formulas

Cardiovascular

Cardiac output
- Cardiac output = heart rate + stroke volume

Mean arterial pressure (MAP)
- MAP = (2/3 diastolic pressure) + (1/3 systolic pressure)
- MAP = cardiac output $\times$ total peripheral resistance

Fick's equation
- Organ O_2 consumption = $(AO_2 - VO_2)$/total organ blood flow

Poiseuille's equation
- $Q = \pi (\Delta P)r^4/8\, L\eta$

  Q = flow of blood through the lumen of a vessel

  η = viscosity

  L = length of tube

  r = radius (*fourth power!*)

  P = pressure

Starling hypothesis
- Flow = $k[(P_i + O_o) - (P_o + O_i)]$

  Flow = flow of fluid through the walls of the capillary

  k = filtration constant of a vessel wall

  P_i = hydrostatic pressure inside the vessel

  O_o = oncotic pressure outside the vessel

  P_o = hydrostatic pressure outside the vessel

  O_i = oncotic pressure inside the vessel

Pulmonary

Arteriolar-alveolar
(A-a) difference • A-a difference = $(150 - \text{Pa}_{CO_2} \times 1.25) - \text{Pa}_{O_2}$ (simplified)

Minute ventilation ($\dot{V}_E$) • $\dot{V}_E$ = tidal volume $\times$ respiratory rate

Renal

Clearance (C) • C = (urine concentration) $\times$ (urine volume) / (plasma concentration)

Transport Mechanisms

Mechanisms That Do Not Require External Energy

Passive diffusion • Passive diffusion occurs when particles flow down a concentration gradient without need for carrier mechanisms. Fick's law applies:

Rate of diffusion = $-PA(C_{in} - C_{out})$

P   = permeability coefficient

A   = area of the membrane

C_{in} = concentration inside membrane

C_{out} = concentration outside membrane

Coach's hint: *Rate of diffusion is **proportional** to the area and the concentration difference.*

Active diffusion • Active diffusion occurs when particles are carried through a membrane by a **carrier molecule.**

• This often occurs for particles that are too big or polar to flow through membranes by passive diffusion (such as large ions).

• In this case, diffusion may be limited by the availability of carrier molecules and **Michaelis-Menten kinetics** may apply.

Mechanisms That Require External Energy (ATP)

Primary active transport • Primary active transport can move particles against an electrochemical gradient by using the energy in high-energy bonds [adenosine triphosphate (ATP)].

  ○ Na^+/K^+-ATPase pump

  ○ Calcium pump (in sarcoplasmic reticulum)

  ○ K^+/H^+ pump (gastric mucosa)

Secondary active transport • Secondary active transport can move particles against an electrochemical gradient by using another electrochemical gradient. No high-energy bonds are directly consumed in this type of transport.

Second Messenger Signal Transduction Pathways

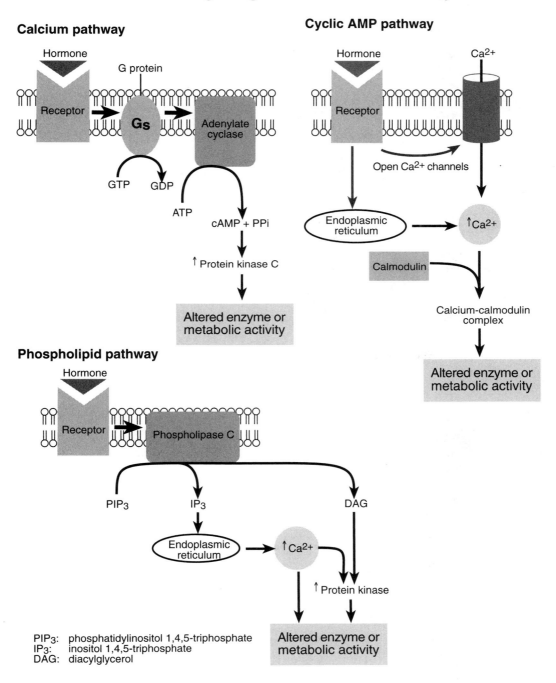

Calcium pathway

Hormone

G protein

Receptor

Gs

Adenylate cyclase

GTP   GDP

ATP

cAMP + PPi

↑ Protein kinase C

Altered enzyme or metabolic activity

Cyclic AMP pathway

Hormone

Ca²⁺

Receptor

Open Ca²⁺ channels

Endoplasmic reticulum

↑Ca²⁺

Calmodulin

Calcium-calmodulin complex

Altered enzyme or metabolic activity

Phospholipid pathway

Hormone

Receptor

Phospholipase C

PIP₃   IP₃   DAG

Endoplasmic reticulum

↑Ca²⁺

↑ Protein kinase

Altered enzyme or metabolic activity

PIP₃: phosphatidylinositol 1,4,5-triphosphate
IP₃: inositol 1,4,5-triphosphate
DAG: diacylglycerol

- Symporters
- Antiporters

Cardiovascular Physiology

Vascular Physiology

Arterioles
- Arterioles are the controlling points (stopcocks) of circulation. Arteriole smooth muscle tone depends on sympathetic input, local metabolites, hormones, and other mediators.

Autoregulation
- Autoregulation maintains a constant blood flow over a wide range of pressures. Constant flow is maintained as a contractile response of vascular smooth muscle either to increases/decreases in pressure (**myogenic theory of autoregulation**) or to increases/decreases in local metabolites (**metabolic theory**).

Venules
- Venules are the most permeable components of the microcirculation.

Endocrine Physiology

Hormone Transport in the Blood
- **Peptide** hormones are hydrophilic and freely dissolve in plasma.

ECG Waveform (highly simplified)

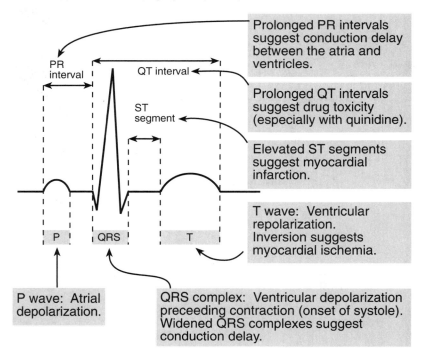

PR interval

QT interval

ST segment

P

QRS

T

Prolonged PR intervals suggest conduction delay between the atria and ventricles.

Prolonged QT intervals suggest drug toxicity (especially with quinidine).

Elevated ST segments suggest myocardial infarction.

T wave: Ventricular repolarization. Inversion suggests myocardial ischemia.

P wave: Atrial depolarization.

QRS complex: Ventricular depolarization preceeding contraction (onset of systole). Widened QRS complexes suggest conduction delay.

Cardiac Action Potential
(Ventricular)

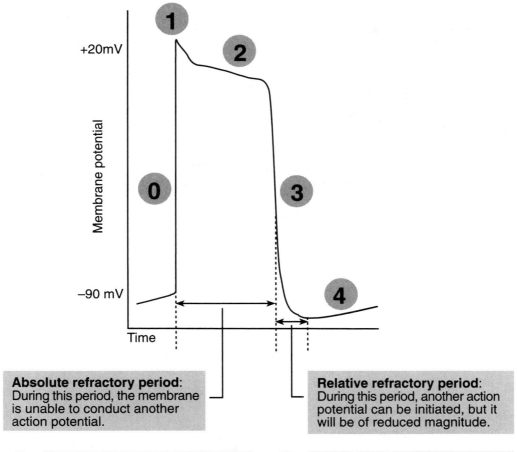

Absolute refractory period: During this period, the membrane is unable to conduct another action potential.

Relative refractory period: During this period, another action potential can be initiated, but it will be of reduced magnitude.

0 **Phase 0:** Rapid depolarization due to opening of voltage-gated Na^+ channels and influx of Na^+.

1 **Phase 1:** Partial repolarization due to a small increase in K^+ permeability. Na^+ channels become inactivated at this time.

2 **Phase 2: Plateau.** This is unique to the cardiac action potential. The plateau is **due to an influx of Ca^{2+}** through the "slow" voltage-gated Ca^{2+} channels. K^+ permeability remains low.

3 **Phase 3:** Rapid repolarization due to inactivation of the Ca^{2+} channels and increase in K^+ permeability. During this time, the Na^+ channels reset, enabling the action potential to be initiated anew.

4 **Phase 4:** Diastolic depolarization due to decreased baseline K^+ permeability. This spontaneous depolarization accounts for the automaticity of cardiac action potentials.

- **Steroid** and **thyroid** hormones are hydrophobic and require plasma proteins to carry them.
  - Some plasma binding proteins, such as thyroid binding globulin, bind only specific hormones; others, such as **albumin,** bind virtually all hormones (as well as other molecules).
  - The total hormone pool is predominantly in bound form; however, **only the free form of hormone is biologically active.**

Anterior Pituitary Gland Hormones

Adrenocorticotropic hormone (ACTH)
- Stimulates cortisol release from the adrenal cortex

Growth hormone (GH)
- Stimulates the growth of bone, cartilage, and connective tissue. After epiphyseal plate fusion, bone lengthening due to GH cannot occur, but bone thickening continues.
- Anabolic effect on skeletal and cardiac muscle leading to **positive nitrogen balance**
- Catabolic effect on adipose tissue
- Diabetogenic effects (anti-insulin effects)

Prolactin
- Stimulates mammary gland development and milk production
- After pregnancy, prolactin stimulates lactose synthesis.
- Suppresses luteinizing hormone (LH) secretion, leading to amenorrhea during lactation

Thyroid-stimulating hormone (TSH)
- Stimulates triiodothyronine (T_3) and thyroxine (T_4) release from the thyroid

Posterior Pituitary Gland Hormones

Antidiuretic hormone (ADH)
- Increases permeability of renal collecting ducts to water, leading to water reabsorption
- Decreases volume and increases osmolarity of urine
- Decreases blood flow to the renal medulla
- Stimulates release of ACTH from the anterior pituitary

Oxytocin
- Stimulates uterine contractions during labor
- Stimulates myoepithelial cells of the mammary gland to contract and causes milk letdown

| Important Points | • | Antidiuretic hormone is released from the **supraoptic nucleus** and is a potent vasoconstrictor. |

Important Points

• Antidiuretic hormone is released from the **supraoptic nucleus** and is a potent vasoconstrictor.

• Oxytocin is released from the **paraventricular nucleus.** Oxytocin causes ejection of milk from the breasts and uterine contractions.

• These hormones are **neural hormones,** meaning that they are secreted by neurons. The neuronal bodies reside in the supraoptic and paraventricular nuclei in the **hypothalamus,** but the nerve endings that release the hormones are located in the posterior lobe of the pituitary.

Thyroid Gland Hormones

Thyroid hormone

• Increases basal metabolic rate of most cells in the body and increases the activity of Na^+K^+-ATPase pumps

• Necessary for normal bone growth and maturation, normal brain maturation, and normal lactation

Calcitonin

• Secreted by the parafollicular cells of the thyroid gland

• Inhibits bone resorption by osteoclasts and osteocytes

• Inhibits gastric motility and gastrin secretion

• Prevents absorption of Ca^{2+} and PO_4^{3-} in jejunum

• Stimulates excretion of Ca^{2+}, Na^{2+}, and phosphate in the kidneys

• Decreases calcitriol synthesis by inhibiting 1α-hydroxylase

• Overall, results in **hypocalcemia** secondary to increased Ca^{2+} uptake into bone

Mnemonic: *Think "calcitonin is calcium to in" (i.e., calcium gets taken out of the bloodstream "into" the bone).*

Important Points

• During thyroid hormone synthesis, thyroid follicular cells become columnar rather than cuboidal in shape.

• The thyroid cell actively transports iodide into the cell against an electrochemical gradient. The iodide then diffuses into the colloid.

• T_4 and T_3 are synthesized in colloid by iodination and condensation of tyrosine molecules bound in peptide linkage to thyroglobulin. The hormones remain bound to thyroglobulin until they are excreted.

• T_3 very significantly and rapidly increases the basal metabolic rate, but its effect diminishes quickly.

• T_4 more weakly and slowly increases basal metabolic rate, and its effect lasts longer.

Thyroid Feedback Inhibition

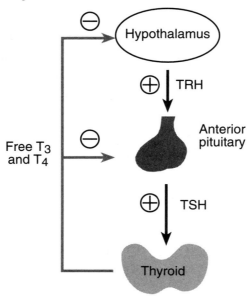

Parathyroid Gland Hormones

Parathyroid hormone (PTH)

- Overall osteolytic effect by stimulating osteoclastic and osteocytic activity while suppressing osteoblastic activity. This release of Ca^{2+} and PO_4^{3-} from bone may cause **hypercalcemia.**
- Acts together with calcitrol to increase intestinal absorption of Ca^{2+} and phosphate
- Stimulates absorption of Ca^{2+} in the distal nephron, but inhibits Ca^{2+} absorption in proximal tubule
- Inhibits phosphate reabsorption in the proximal tubule, leading to **hypophosphatemia**
- Increases calcitriol synthesis by stimulating 1α-hydroxylase activity
- Increases renal excretion of Na^+, K^+, and HCO_{3-}

Pancreatic Hormones

Insulin

- Promotes storage and utilization of glucose (glycolysis)
- Stimulates amino acid uptake and protein synthesis in muscle cells
- Stimulates fatty acid and triglyceride synthesis and inhibits lipolysis in adipose cells

Calcium Regulation

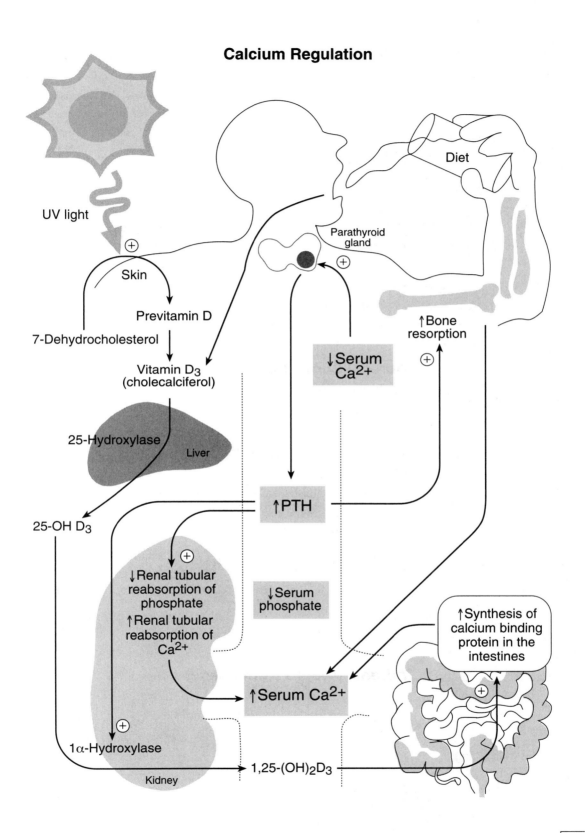

UV light

Skin

7-Dehydrocholesterol

Previtamin D

Vitamin D$_3$
(cholecalciferol)

25-Hydroxylase

Liver

25-OH D$_3$

Diet

Parathyroid
gland

$\oplus$

$\downarrow$Serum
Ca^{2+}

$\uparrow$Bone
resorption

$\oplus$

$\uparrow$PTH

$\oplus$
$\downarrow$Renal tubular
reabsorption of
phosphate
$\uparrow$Renal tubular
reabsorption of
Ca^{2+}

$\downarrow$Serum
phosphate

$\uparrow$Synthesis of
calcium binding
protein in the
intestines

$\uparrow$Serum Ca^{2+}

$\oplus$

$\oplus$
1α-Hydroxylase

Kidney

1,25-(OH)$_2$D$_3$

- Stimulates lipogenesis and inhibits proteolysis in the liver
- Lowers serum K^+ concentration by stimulating increased uptake in muscle and adipose tissue
- The uptake of glucose by the brain, erythrocytes, and liver is **independent of insulin.**

Glucagon
- Stimulates hepatic glycogenolysis
- Promotes gluconeogenesis

Somatostatin
- Inhibits thyrotropin and GH secretion in the anterior pituitary
- Inhibits glucagon, insulin, and pancreatic polypeptide secretion in pancreas
- Inhibits digestion by inhibiting secretion of gut hormones, gastric acid, and pepsin, as well as by decreasing gut blood flow and motility

Adrenal Cortex Hormones

Aldosterone
- Increases Na^+ reabsorption in the distal convoluted tubules in the kidneys

Cortisol
- Anti-inflammatory effects
- Stress adaptation
- Stimulates gluconeogenesis, blocks uptake of glucose in tissues, and inhibits glycolytic enzymes
- Mobilizes fatty acids from adipose tissue to the liver and stimulates lipolysis
- Increases release of amino acids from skeletal muscle and other tissues while inhibiting protein synthesis. This leads to **negative nitrogen balance.**

Adrenal Medulla Hormones

Epinephrine, norepinephrine
- Sympathetic effects on target organs
- Elevate blood glucose

Adrenal Gland
Hormone Production

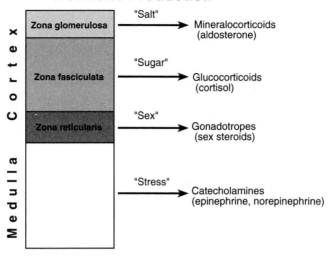

Zona glomerulosa	"Salt" →	Mineralocorticoids (aldosterone)	
Zona fasciculata	"Sugar" →	Glucocorticoids (cortisol)	
Zona reticularis	"Sex" →	Gonadotropes (sex steroids)	
	"Stress" →	Catecholamines (epinephrine, norepinephrine)	

Cortisol Feedback Inhibition

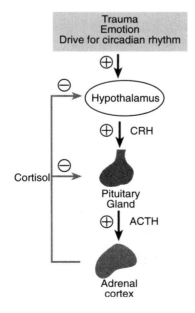

Steroid Synthesis

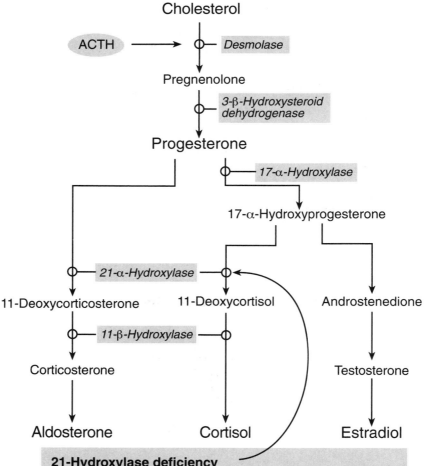

Cholesterol

ACTH ⟶ ⊖ *Desmolase*

Pregnenolone

⊖ *3-β-Hydroxysteroid dehydrogenase*

Progesterone

⊖ *17-α-Hydroxylase*

17-α-Hydroxyprogesterone

⊖ *21-α-Hydroxylase* ⊖

11-Deoxycorticosterone   11-Deoxycortisol   Androstenedione

⊖ *11-β-Hydroxylase* ⊖

Corticosterone   Testosterone

Aldosterone   Cortisol   Estradiol

21-Hydroxylase deficiency

- 21-Hydroxylase deficiency is the most common steroid enzyme defect.
- Loss of this enzyme results in shunting of steroid synthesis to androgen and estrogen generation. Patients therefore have defects in cortisol and mineralocorticoid synthesis, and have elevated androgen and ACTH levels.
- Female infants with this deficiency have ambiguous or male genitalia but no testicles.

Adrenal Insufficiency

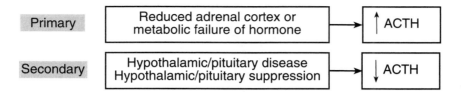

Primary → Reduced adrenal cortex or metabolic failure of hormone → ↑ ACTH

Secondary → Hypothalamic/pituitary disease Hypothalamic/pituitary suppression → ↓ ACTH

Kidney Hormones

Renin
- Renin release is stimulated by a drop in serum Na^+ and a decrease in blood flow to the kidneys
- Converts angiotensinogen to angiotensin I

Calcitriol
- 1,25-Dihydroxyvitamin D_3
- Works synergistically with PTH to increase absorption of Ca^{2+} and phosphate in the small intestine

Renin-Angiotensin-Aldosterone System

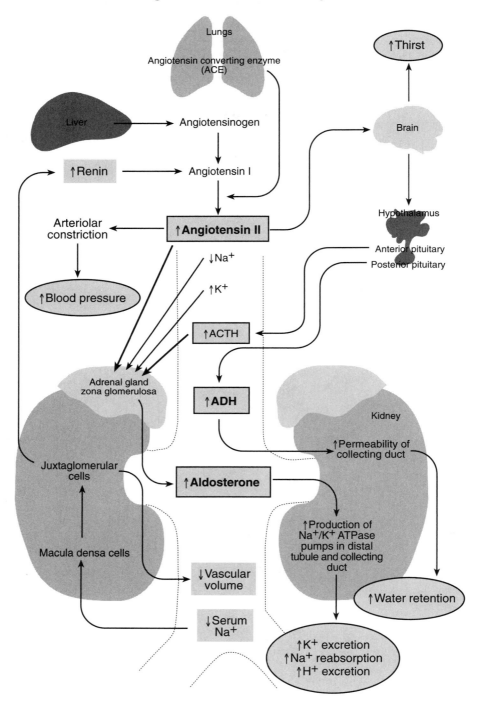

Renal Tubule Physiology

Most diuretics enter the renal tubule through the acid secretion system in the proximal tubule and can cause it to saturate. This is why certain patients develop **hyperuricemia** on loop or thiazide diuretics.

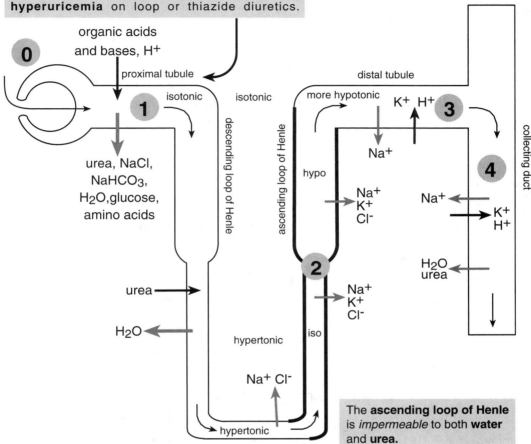

The **ascending loop of Henle** is *impermeable* to both **water** and **urea**.

0 **Mannitol:** osmotic diuretic; works throughout the nephron

1 **Acetazolamide:** carbonic anhydrase inhibitor with weak diuretic properties; prevents the exchange of H^+ and Na^+

2 **Furosemide, bumetanide, ethacrynic acid:** most effective diuretics; inhibit $Na^+/K^+/Cl^-$ cotransport from the ascending loop of Henle; this results in increased excretion of Na^+, K^+, Cl^-, and water

3 **Thiazide diuretics:** work by inibiting Na^+ and Cl^- reabsorption in the distal convoluted tubule

Aldosterone: acts on the distal tubule cells to actively reabsorb Na^+ — this results in the passive secretion of K^+

Spironolactone, amiloride, triamterene: inhibits the action of aldosterone, preventing the reabsorption of Na^+ and the secretion of K^+; these are **potassium sparing diuretics**

4 **Antidiuretic hormone (ADH):** increases the permeability of renal cells in the **distal tubule and collecting duct** to water; this results in increased reabsorption and retention of water

Parietal Cell Control

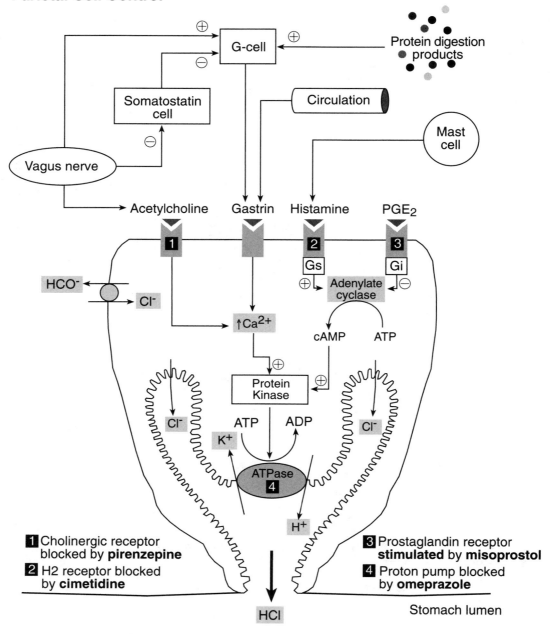

1 Cholinergic receptor blocked by **pirenzepine**
2 H2 receptor blocked by **cimetidine**
3 Prostaglandin receptor stimulated by **misoprostol**
4 Proton pump blocked by **omeprazole**

Arachidonic Acid Metabolites

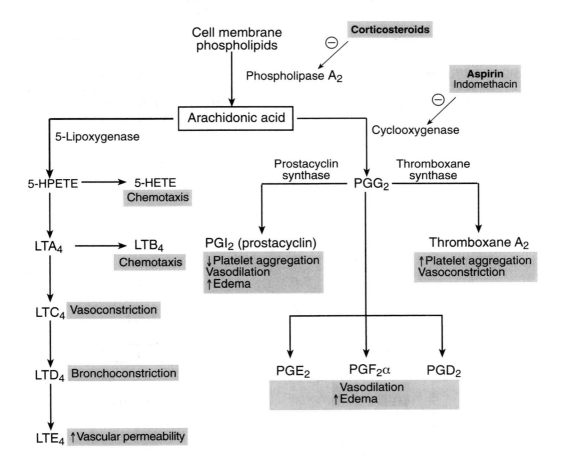

Menstrual cycle
(Classic 28-day cycle)

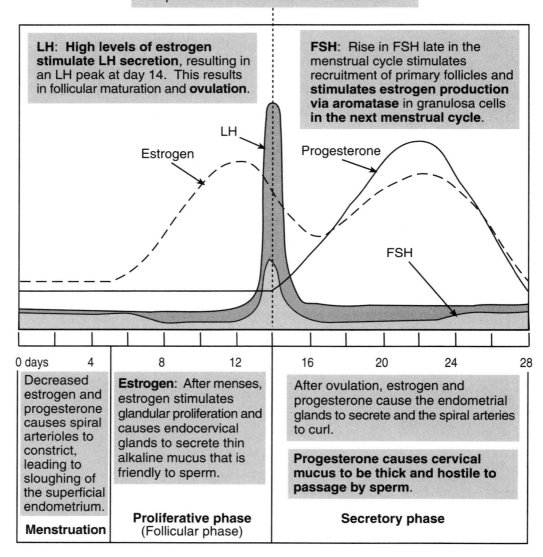

Ovulation (day 14): The egg completes the first meiotic division just before ovulation. The resulting secondary oocyte then begins the second meiotic division **up to metaphase II**. If this oocyte is fertilized, then it will go on to complete the second meiotic division.

LH: **High levels of estrogen stimulate LH secretion**, resulting in an LH peak at day 14. This results in follicular maturation and **ovulation**.

FSH: Rise in FSH late in the menstrual cycle stimulates recruitment of primary follicles and **stimulates estrogen production via aromatase** in granulosa cells **in the next menstrual cycle**.

Estrogen

LH

Progesterone

FSH

0 days   4   8   12   16   20   24   28

Decreased estrogen and progesterone causes spiral arterioles to constrict, leading to sloughing of the superficial endometrium.

Menstruation

Estrogen: After menses, estrogen stimulates glandular proliferation and causes endocervical glands to secrete thin alkaline mucus that is friendly to sperm.

Proliferative phase
(Follicular phase)

After ovulation, estrogen and progesterone cause the endometrial glands to secrete and the spiral arteries to curl.

Progesterone causes cervical mucus to be thick and hostile to passage by sperm.

Secretory phase

Anatomy

CHAPTER 7

Erich S. Huang

_____ **Coach's Tips**

- Anatomy is a low-yield subject. Nevertheless, there are several points to be gained. For this reason, we present a concise but detailed section that covers many anatomy questions on the Boards.
- Computerized tomogram (CT) cross-sectional anatomy and electron micrographs are tested.
- Neuroanatomic pathways and major limb nerves are high yield.
- **Major** vessels and important smaller arteries, such as the middle cerebral and middle meningeal, are high yield.
- Muscles are low yield.

_____ **Microanatomy**

Cell Junctions and
Junctional Complexes •
- **Tight junctions,** also called zona occludens, are small areas just below the luminal surface of cells where layers of opposing plasma membranes are fused to one another. In watertight epithelia, such as the urinary bladder or intestinal mucosa, these junctions are plentiful and form an impermeable belt around each cell. In other tissues, tight junctions are more sparse.
- **Adherent junctions,** also called zona adherens, are found just deep to tight junctions. These structures form a uniform space between opposing plasma membranes and also form a belt around each cell. They are thought to be important for anchoring the microfilaments and actin in intestinal microvilli.
- **Desmosomes,** also called macula adherens, are electron dense anchoring points just below the adherent junctions. Desmosomes are anchored to the cytoplasm by tonofilaments and help dissipate physical forces at the attachment sites. They are plentiful in epithelial cells that are subject to abrasion and physical stress.
- **Gap junctions** are special groups of channels between cells that allow for rapid and direct movement of molecules and action potentials from cell to cell. These round, plate-like plasma membrane ad-

hesions are studded with numerous ion channels. The ion channels span a very narrow intercellular space.

Epithelia
- Epithelium can be simple or stratified. In other words, arranged in single or multi-layers of cells.

Simple epithelium
- **Squamous epithelium** consists of flattened cells to facilitate rapid diffusion of gases. Simple squamous epithelium defines the alveolae and the luminal surfaces of blood and lymph vessels.
- **Cuboidal epithelium** is specialized for secretion. It lines secretory organs such as tubules in the salivary glands, reproductive tract, and kidney.
- **Columnar epithelium** differs from cuboidal in that columnar epithelium is specialized for both secretion and absorption. It lines the gastrointestinal (GI) tract and often forms microvilli in order to increase absorptive surface area on luminal surfaces.
- **Pseudostratified columnar epithelium** is distinguished by apical cilia and a stratified appearance due to the location of nuclei both apically and basally. All cells contact the basement membrane and therefore consist of a monolayer. It lines tracts requiring ciliary motion, including the trachea and the fallopian tubes.

Stratified epithelium
- **Stratified squamous epithelium** is composed of multiple layers, with germinal cells toward the basement membrane and keratinized cells toward the surface. This specialized epithelium withstands abrasion on areas such as the skin, esophagus, mouth, anus, and vagina.
- **Transitional epithelium** consists of multiple layers of "pillowy" cells. It lines organs that undergo frequent distention and contraction such as the urinary bladder and ureters.

Histologic Stains

Hematoxylin and Eosin (H&E) Stains
- Hematoxylin (H) is blue and basophilic. It stains negatively charged structures such as DNA and RNA.
- Eosin (E) is pink and acidophilic. It stains positively charged structures such as mitochondria.
- The Golgi apparatus consists mainly of lipid and remains unstained.

- Iron hematoxylin stains secretory granules black.
- Periodic acid-Schiff (PAS) stains glycogen magenta.
- Naturally occurring brown pigments include the skin pigment melanin, the aging pigment lipofuscin, and hemosiderin, which accumulates in macrophages after an old hemorrhage.

Gross Anatomy

**Cross Sectional
Anatomy**

- Cross-sectional anatomy is fair game on the Boards.

Cross Sectional Anatomy: Chest

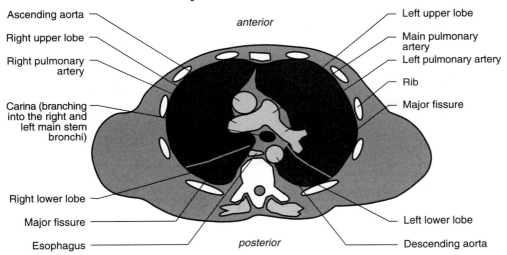

Ascending aorta

anterior

Left upper lobe

Right upper lobe

Main pulmonary artery

Right pulmonary artery

Left pulmonary artery

Rib

Carina (branching into the right and left main stem bronchi)

Major fissure

Right lower lobe

Left lower lobe

Major fissure

Esophagus

posterior

Descending aorta

Cross Sectional Anatomy: Abdomen

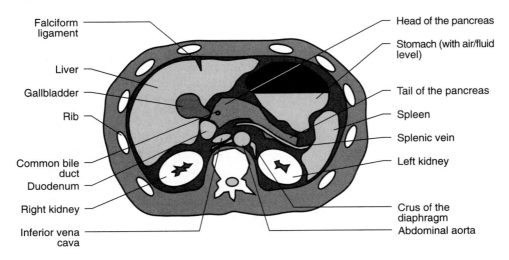

Falciform ligament

Head of the pancreas

Liver

Stomach (with air/fluid level)

Gallbladder

Tail of the pancreas

Rib

Spleen

Splenic vein

Common bile duct

Left kidney

Duodenum

Right kidney

Crus of the diaphragm

Inferior vena cava

Abdominal aorta

Common Procedures and Anatomic Landmarks

Thoracentesis
- Insert the needle **just over rib 9**, not under rib 8, or you could puncture the intercostal vein, artery, or nerve.
- The inferior edge of the scapula lies over the 7th intercostal space.
- Complication: Pneumothorax.

Lumbar Puncture
- Insert the needle between L3 and L5.
- The iliac crest marks L4.
- **The needle does not penetrate pia mater.** CSF can be withdrawn when the subarachnoid space is entered.
- Complications: Headache, herniation, and epidural/subdural hematomas.

Gluteal Injections
- Upper outer quadrant of hip.
- Avoid the sciatic nerve. **Injury to the sciatic can result in footdrop.**

Abdominal Wall Layers
1) Skin
2) Subcutaneous tissue
3) Superficial Scarpa's fascia
4) External oblique
5) Internal oblique
6) Transversus abdominis
7) Transversalis fascia
8) Preperitoneal fat and areolar tissue
9) Peritoneum

Common Bony Injuries

Wrist Fractures
- **Colles' fractures** are fractures of the distal radius caused by falling onto an outstretched hand.
- **Scaphoid fractures** are the most common carpal bone fracture.

Clavicular Fracture
- The **clavicle is the most frequently fractured bone**, and may be fractured during birth trauma.
- Complications: brachial nerve palsy, usually Erb's type ("waiter's tip"). This nerve injury is characterized by shoulder medial rotation, forearm pronation, and arm hanging by the patient's side.

Hip Dislocation
- Posterior dislocation is most common.
- This dislocation internally rotates, adducts, and flexes the leg at the hip.
- Complications: **avascular necrosis**, late traumatic arthritis, and sciatic nerve injury

Femoral Neck Fractures
- These result from falls, **commonly in elderly women**.
- In young active patients, **stress fractures** are the most common etiology. These patients may remain ambulatory.
- Symptoms include pain in the groin and medial leg, loss of hip motion, and pain with rotation.
- **Patients are at high risk for avascular necrosis of the femoral neck**.

Knee
- A lateral blow to the knee damages the medial collateral ligament, medial meniscus, and anterior cruciate ligament.
- Lateral collateral ligament injury is rare.

Peripheral Neuroanatomy

Innervation and Action of Nerves

Radial nerve (C5-8)
- Extends the elbow and wrist
- Triceps reflex

Median nerve (C6-T1)
- Flexes the first three fingers
- Mediates pronator and radial flexion
- Innervates the thenar muscles controlling thumb opposition

Ulnar nerve (C8-T1)
- Adducts the thumb
- Flexes the wrist and ring and small finger
- Opposition of little finger
- Mediates ulnar flexion
- Abducts and adducts the fingers
- Innervates the hypothenar muscles

Musculocutaneous nerve (C5-6)
- Flexes the elbow (biceps)
- Supinates (biceps)
- Biceps reflex

Axillary nerve (C5-6)
- Moves the arm outward, forward, or backwards (deltoids)

Long thoracic nerve (C5-7)
- Elevates the arm above horizontal

Femoral nerve (L2-4)
- Extends the knee
- Flexes the hip
- Knee jerk reflex

Obturator nerve (L2-4)
- Adducts the hip

Sciatic nerve (L4-S3)
- Flexes the knee
- Branches into the tibial and common peroneal nerves

Tibial nerve (L4-S3)
- Inverts the foot
- Flexes the foot downward (plantar flexion)
- Ankle jerk reflex

Common peroneal nerve (L4-S2)
- Everts the foot
- Flexes the foot up (dorsiflexion)

Nerve Injuries

Long thoracic nerve

- Innervates serratus anterior muscle
- Results in **winged scapula** (posterior protrusion of scapula with forward pushing of the arms)
- Suggests brachial plexus injury relatively close to vertebral column

Ulnar nerve

- Injury results in ulnar **claw hand,** inability to adduct fingers secondary to interosseous paralysis
- Sensory deficits of dorsal and palmar aspects of 4th and 5th digits

Brachial plexus

- Results in severe claw hand that resembles an **L** because of [**L**]umbrical paralysis and impaired wrist flexion
- Impairs the median and ulnar nerves
- Sensory deficits along C8-T1 dermatomes
- Injury may result from cervical rib compression, sudden arm traction, birth injury, or compression from lymph node metastases.

Common peroneal nerve

- Results in **footdrop**—inability to evert and dorsiflex foot
- Injured by blows to lateral posterior knee, classically by a briefcase or bowling ball

Carpal tunnel syndrome

- Results from **median nerve** compression in the carpal tunnel at the wrist
- Symptoms include numbness and tingling of the hand and thumb.
- May be secondary to repetitive motion
- Women are affected twice as commonly as men.

Central Neuroanatomy

Thalamus

The thalamus is part of the diencephalon. It has seven major nuclei, including:

Mediodorsal nucleus

- This nucleus is involved in limbic function. Destruction results in memory loss (such as in Wernicke-Korsakoff syndrome). Note that Wernicke-Korsakoff syndrome also involves lesions of the mammillary bodies.

Lateral geniculate nucleus

- This nucleus is involved in the relay of visual stimuli.

Medial geniculate nucleus

- This nucleus is involved in the relay of auditory stimuli.

	Cortical Region	Deficit
Frontal Lobe	Motor/premotor cortex	Contralateral spastic paralysis
	Broca's area	Nonfluent aphasia with inability to produce speech (understands language but cannot speak or write); also called expressive aphasia
		*Mnemonic: Damage to **Bro**ca's area in the **Bro**ntal lobe results in inability to **bro**duce speech.*
	Prefrontal cortex	Loss of judgment and abstracting abilities
Parietal Lobe	Sensory cortex	Destruction results in contralateral hypoesthesia and astereognosis
	Superior parietal lobule	Contralateral astereognosis and sensory **neglect**
Temporal Lobe	Primary auditory cortex	Unilateral destruction—slight hearing loss Bilateral destruction—cortical deafness
	Wernicke's area	Fluent aphasia with inability to receive and understand speech; also called receptive aphasia
		*Mnemonic: Damage to **We**rnicke's area results in inability to **We**ceive or **We**cognize speech.*
	Hippocampus	Bilateral lesions result in inability to form new memories
	Anterior temporal lobe	Bilateral damage to the amygdala results in Klüver-Bucy syndrome (hypersexuality, visual agnosia, hyperphagia, and docility)

Other Important Lesions

- **Argyll Robertson pupil** is secondary to **syphilis.** The affected pupil accommodates but does not react. Lesion is in the pretectal region of the superior colliculus.
- **Pituitary tumors** compress the optic chiasm, resulting in **bitemporal hemianopsia.** If a pituitary tumor (or one nearby) is **calcified,** it is probably a **craniopharyngioma.**

Anatomy and Disorders of the Basal Ganglia

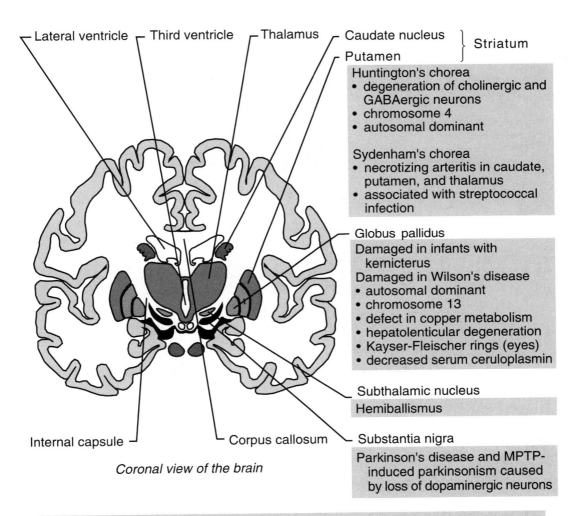

Lateral ventricle — Third ventricle — Thalamus — Caudate nucleus ⎫
Putamen ⎬ Striatum

Huntington's chorea
- degeneration of cholinergic and GABAergic neurons
- chromosome 4
- autosomal dominant

Sydenham's chorea
- necrotizing arteritis in caudate, putamen, and thalamus
- associated with streptococcal infection

Globus pallidus
Damaged in infants with kernicterus
Damaged in Wilson's disease
- autosomal dominant
- chromosome 13
- defect in copper metabolism
- hepatolenticular degeneration
- Kayser-Fleischer rings (eyes)
- decreased serum ceruloplasmin

Subthalamic nucleus
Hemiballismus

Substantia nigra
Parkinson's disease and MPTP-induced parkinsonism caused by loss of dopaminergic neurons

Internal capsule — Corpus callosum

Coronal view of the brain

- The **basal ganglia** generally refers to the caudate nucleus, putamen, and globus pallidus and the subthalamic nucleus and substantia nigra.
- The caudate nucleus and putamen are sometimes called the **striatum**.
- The putamen and globus pallidus are sometimes called the **lenticular nucleus**.

Spinal Cord Cross-section

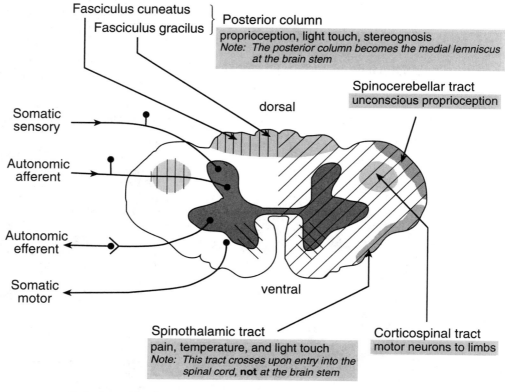

Fasciculus cuneatus
Fasciculus gracilus
} Posterior column
proprioception, light touch, stereognosis
Note: The posterior column becomes the medial lemniscus at the brain stem

Spinocerebellar tract
unconscious proprioception

dorsal

Somatic sensory

Autonomic afferent

Autonomic efferent

Somatic motor

ventral

Spinothalamic tract
pain, temperature, and light touch
*Note: This tract crosses upon entry into the spinal cord, **not** at the brain stem*

Corticospinal tract
motor neurons to limbs

Spinal cord lesions

	Disease	Affected area of the spinal cord
	Syringomyelia	Bilateral involvement of the ventral horns
	Pernicious anemia	Dorsal columns and corticospinal tract
	Brown-Séquard syndrome	Hemisection of the spinal cord

Neurotransmitters

- **Acetylcholine** is the major neurotransmitter of the peripheral nervous system (PNS). Loss of acetylcholine through degeneration of the basal nucleus of Meynert is associated with Alzheimer's disease.

- **Catecholamines**
  - **Epinephrine:** generated predominantly by the adrenal medulla
  - **Dopamine:** depleted in Parkinson's disease (D1 receptors); excessive in schizophrenia (D2 receptors)
  - **Norepinephrine:** The **catecholamine hypothesis** proposes that excess of norepinephrine is involved in mania, and deficiency is involved in depression.

Flow of CSF

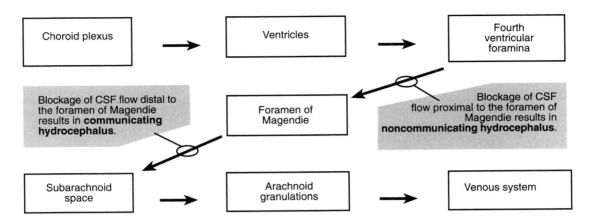

- **Serotonin**
    - ○ Low levels allow decreased levels of catecholamines to cause mood disorders.
    - ○ Many antidepressants, including fluoxetine, inhibit serotonin re-uptake.
    - ○ High levels of serotonin may thus help stabilize mood.
- **γ-Aminobutyric acid (GABA):** the major inhibitory neurotransmitter of the central nervous system (CNS)
- **Glycine:** the major inhibitory neurotransmitter of the PNS
- **Glutamate:** the major excitatory neurotransmitter of the CNS

Embryology

CHAPTER 8

Kevin Courtney

Coach's Tips

- Embryology is moderate yield at best. We provide an overview for those who do not have time to read extensively.
- Pharyngeal pouch derivatives, branchial arch derivatives, and branchial cleft derivatives are high yield.

Principal Branchial Derivatives

Groove	Arch	Pouch
I Pinna and external auditory meatus	Mandible, malleus, incus, anterior tongue, m. of mastication, tensors tympani and veli palatini m., mylohyoid m., ant. belly digastric m., trigeminal nerve	Auditory tube, middle ear cavity
II	Lesser horns of hyoid, styloid process, stapes, m. of facial expression, stapedius m., stylohyoid m., facial nerve	Tonsillar fossa
III	Greater horns of hyoid, stylopharyngeus m., posterior tongue, glossopharyngeal nerve	Thymus, inferior parathyroids
IV	Thyroid cartilage, cricothyroid m., posterior tongue, superior laryngeal nerve	Superior parathyroids
V	N/A	Perifollicular cells of thyroid
VI	Cricoid and arytenoid cartilages, intrinsic laryngeal m., inferior laryngeal nerve	Laryngeal ventricle

Adult Derivatives of the Pharyngeal Pouches and Branchial Arches and Grooves

(Correlate with table below)

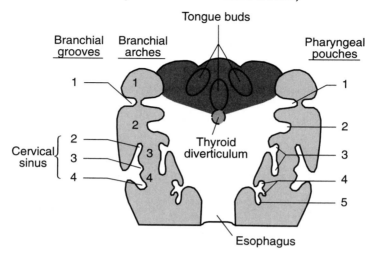

Horizontal section at 5 weeks

Malformations

Cleft Lip
- Results from incomplete fusion of the maxillary prominence with the median nasal prominence.

Cleft Palate
- Results from incomplete fusion of the lateral palatine processes with each other, with the median nasal septum, and/or with the median palatine process.
- Cleft lip with or without cleft palate is the classic example of multi-factorial inheritance.

Principal Aortic Arch Derivatives

Arch	Derivative
I	Maxillary arteries and external carotid arteries
II	Stapedial arteries
III Proximal	**Common carotid arteries**
III Distal	**Internal carotid arteries**
IV Left	Aortic arch: Aortic sac gives rise to **proximal aortic arch.** Left dorsal aorta gives rise to **distal aortic arch**
IV Right	Proximal **right subclavian artery**

continued

Arch	Derivative
V	Rudimentary vessels
VI Left	Proximal left pulmonary artery
	Ductus arteriosus
VI Right	Proximal right pulmonary artery

Fetal Circulation

- The figure following illustrates fetal circulation.
- Richly oxygenated blood is supplied by the placenta through the **umbilical vein.**
- Blood with low oxygen tension returns from the fetus to the placenta through two **umbilical arteries.**

Fetal Structure	Neonatal Derivative
Ductus arteriosus	Ligamentum arteriosum
Foramen ovale	Fossa ovalis
Ductus venosus	Ligamentum venosum
Umbilical vein	Ligamentum teres

Heart

Development of the Heart

- The heart develops as a simple endothelial tube.
- In the developing embryo, angioblastic cords form, become canalized, and result in the two endothelial heart tubes. These two tubes eventually fuse to form a single endothelial tube.

Compartmentalization of the Heart

- The tubular heart forms the truncus arteriosus, bulbus cordis, primitive ventricle, primitive atrium, and sinus venosus. This process coincides with the folding of the embryonic head.
- **The cardiovascular system is the first functioning system in the developing embryo. The myocardium begins contracting on day 21 or 22.**
- **The primitive heart undergoes partitioning by the middle of the fourth week and is completely partitioned by the end of the fifth week.**

Endocardial cushions
- *Endocardial cushions* are swellings of the walls of the atrioventricular canal that approach each other and fuse, forming a septum between the primitive atrium and the primitive ventricle.

Fetal Circulation

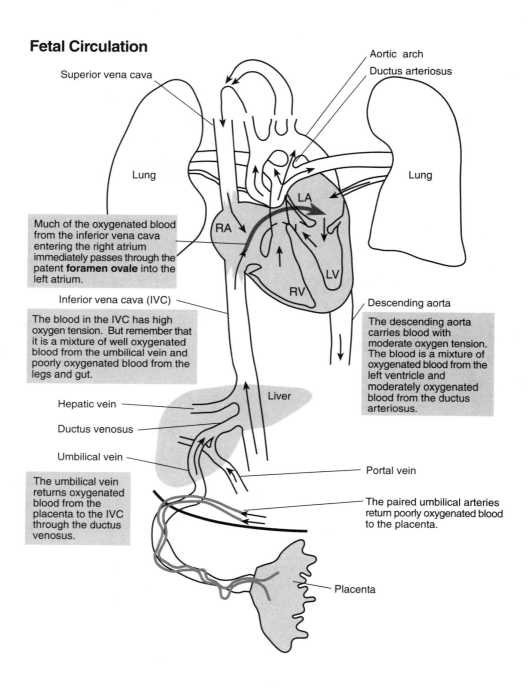

Superior vena cava

Aortic arch

Ductus arteriosus

Lung

Lung

LA

RA

Much of the oxygenated blood from the inferior vena cava entering the right atrium immediately passes through the patent **foramen ovale** into the left atrium.

LV

RV

Inferior vena cava (IVC)

Descending aorta

The blood in the IVC has high oxygen tension. But remember that it is a mixture of well oxygenated blood from the umbilical vein and poorly oxygenated blood from the legs and gut.

The descending aorta carries blood with moderate oxygen tension. The blood is a mixture of oxygenated blood from the left ventricle and moderately oxygenated blood from the ductus arteriosus.

Liver

Hepatic vein

Ductus venosus

Umbilical vein

Portal vein

The umbilical vein returns oxygenated blood from the placenta to the IVC through the ductus venosus.

The paired umbilical arteries return poorly oxygenated blood to the placenta.

Placenta

Development of the Heart

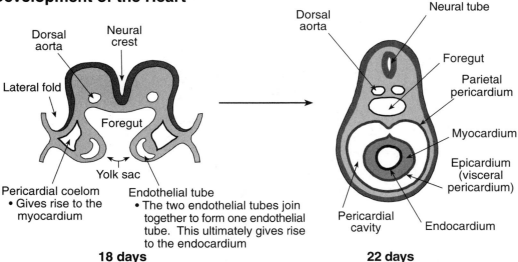

18 days

Dorsal aorta

Neural crest

Lateral fold

Foregut

Yolk sac

Pericardial coelom
• Gives rise to the myocardium

Endothelial tube
• The two endothelial tubes join together to form one endothelial tube. This ultimately gives rise to the endocardium

22 days

Dorsal aorta

Neural tube

Foregut

Parietal pericardium

Myocardium

Epicardium (visceral pericardium)

Endocardium

Pericardial cavity

Primitive atrium
: • The *primitive atrium* is divided into the right and left atria by the formation and fusion of the **septum primum** and **septum secundum.** The septum secundum is incomplete, leaving an oval opening called the **foramen ovale.** The septum primum acts as a flap-like valve covering the foramen ovale, allowing blood to flow from the right atrium to the left atrium but not vice versa. After birth, this region normally seals off to form the **fossa ovalis.**

Coronary sinus
: • The *coronary sinus* arises from the left horn of the **sinus venosus,** and part of the right atrium arises from the right horn of the sinus venosus.

Primitive ventricle
: • The *primitive ventricle* is divided into the left and right ventricles by the formation and growth of the **interventricular septum.** The inferior bulboventricular ridge forms the muscular portion of the septum, and the endocardial cushions form the membranous component of the interventricular septum.

Bulbus cordis
: • The *bulbus cordis* gets incorporated into the left and right ventricles. In the left ventricle, the bulbus cordis gives rise to the opening of the aorta. In the right ventricle, the bulbus cordis becomes the **conus arteriosus** or **infundibulum,** and gives rise to the pulmonary trunks.

Truncus arteriosus
: • The *truncus arteriosus* divides into the aortic and pulmonary trunks by forming the **aorticopulmonary** or **spiral septum.**

Sagittal View of the Primitive Heart at 24 Days

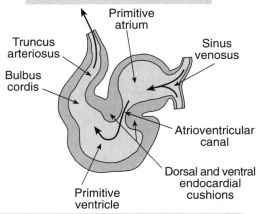

Blood enters the aortic sac and is distributed in the aortic arches

Primitive atrium

Truncus arteriosus

Sinus venosus

Bulbus cordis

Atrioventricular canal

Dorsal and ventral endocardial cushions

Primitive ventricle

Blood enters the sinus venosus from the common cardinal, umbilical, and vitelline veins

Development of the Right and Left Atrium

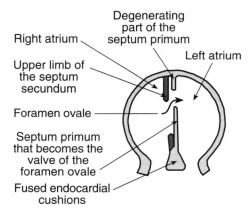

Degenerating part of the septum primum

Right atrium

Left atrium

Upper limb of the septum secundum

Foramen ovale

Septum primum that becomes the valve of the foramen ovale

Fused endocardial cushions

Congenital Defects of the Heart

Ventricular Septal Defects (VSDs)
- VSDs are the most common congenital heart defect.

Membranous VSD
- Most common VSD.
- Results from incomplete closure of the interventricular foramen by the endocardial cushions.

Common Ventricle
- Results from the absence of the interventricular septum.
- Most cases present with transposition of the great vessels.

Atrial Septal Defects (ASDs)
- ASDs and patent ductus arteriosus are the second and third most common congenital cardiac defects.

Patent Foramen Ovale
- The most common heart *anomaly* (*not* defect).
- An isolated patent foramen ovale is of no hemodynamic significance.
- A patent foramen ovale becomes significant only when coupled with other defects (e.g., pulmonary atresia). The resulting right-to-left shunt leads to cyanosis.

Secundum ASD
- Caused by defects in the septum primum and septum secundum in the area of the fossa ovalis.

Sinus Venosus ASD
- Located close to the entry of the superior vena cava.
- Results from incomplete incorporation of the sinus venosus into the right atrium.

Endocardial Cushion/ Atrioventricular (AV) Septal Defect with Primum ASD
- Occurs when the septum primum does not fuse with the endocardial cushions, resulting in a patent foramen primum.
- In 20% of persons with **Down's syndrome,** the endocardial cushions fail to fuse. An AV septal defect results.

Patent Ductus Arteriosus
- Kept open in the fetus by prostaglandins. These prostaglandins are produced in response to low oxygen tension in blood passing through the ductus arteriosus.
- Almost universal in premature infants < 1750 g.
- Treated with indomethacin to inhibit prostaglandin synthesis.

Abnormal Division of the Truncus Arteriosus

Tetralogy of Fallot
- The four defects are:
  1) Ventricular septal defect
  2) Overriding aorta
  3) Pulmonary stenosis
  4) Hypertrophy of the right ventricle

Persistence of the
Truncus Arteriosus
- Incomplete formation of the aorticopulmonary septum results in a single vessel giving rise to both the aorta and pulmonary trunk.

Transposition of the
Great Vessels
- The most common cause of cyanotic heart disease in newborns.
- Results from incomplete spiraling during partitioning of the truncus arteriosus.

Lungs

- The lung bud develops from the laryngotracheal diverticulum.
- Bronchial buds form primary bronchi. Splanchnic mesoderm covering the buds form the visceral pleura.

Four Stages of Lung Development

- Glandular or pseudoglandular period (**weeks 5 to 17**):
  Conducting bronchioles develop.
- Canalicular period (**weeks 16 to 25**):
  Respiratory bronchioles and primitive alveoli develop.
- Terminal sac period (**weeks 24 to birth**):
  Terminal sacs develop. By the 28th week, lung development is adequate for the survival of premature infants. **Alveolar type II cells produce sufficient surfactant to sustain life as early as 28 weeks.**
- Alveolar period (**late fetal to 8 years**):
  Alveolar ducts and mature alveoli develop.

Defects in Lung Development

- Terminal sac formation is the single most crucial period of development.

- Hyaline membrane disease or respiratory distress syndrome of the newborn is associated with deficiency of **pulmonary surfactant,** occurring most commonly in premature infants.

Gastrointestinal

Foregut

Derivatives
- Foregut derivatives include one third of the oral cavity as well as the oropharynx, esophagus, stomach, upper half of the duodenum, common bile duct, liver, pancreas, and pancreatic ducts.

Vasculature
- Vasculature arises from the celiac artery, branches of the external carotids, and thoracic aorta.

Defects
- Foregut defects result in stenoses or fistulas between the esophagus and trachea, esophageal atresia, duodenal atresia, and hypertrophic pyloric stenosis.

Midgut

Derivatives
- Midgut derivatives include the duodenum below the origin of the common bile duct, jejunum, ileum, cecum, appendix, and the proximal colon up to the splenic flexure.

Vasculature
- Vasculature arises from the superior mesenteric artery.

Defects
- Midgut defects result in omphalocele, malrotation and Meckel's diverticulum. Duodenal and esophageal atresia causes polyhydramnios because the fetus cannot swallow amniotic fluid.

Hindgut

Derivatives
- Hindgut derivatives include the descending colon, sigmoid colon, rectum, and upper two thirds of the anal canal.

Vasculature
- Vasculature arises from the inferior mesenteric artery and middle and inferior rectal arteries.

Defects
- Hindgut defects are anorectal and include fistulas between the rectum and urogenital sinus, imperforate anus, and Hirschsprung's disease.

Liver

- The hepatic diverticulum arises from foregut endoderm. It in turn gives rise to the liver, common bile duct, hepatic duct, cystic duct, and gallbladder.
- **Hematopoiesis** occurs in the fetal liver from the second month until birth.

Kidney

- Intermediate mesoderm gives rise to the **pronephros, mesonephros, and metanephros.**

Pronephros
- The pronephros is the first to appear at cervical levels. Tubules degenerate and ducts remain at lower levels as mesonephric ducts.

Mesonephros
- The mesonephros regresses in females.
- In males, the mesonephroi form genital ducts. The ducts give rise to the ductus epididymis, ductus deferens, seminal vesicle, and ejaculatory duct.

Metanephros
- The metanephros forms the permanent kidney.
- Nephrons arise from the metanephric mesoderm.
  Collecting tubules arise from the metanephric diverticulum.

Kidney Development (week 5)

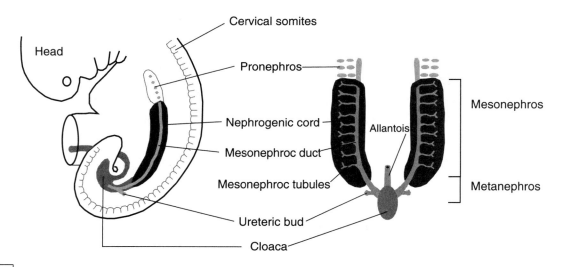

Ectopic kidneys • Ectopic kidneys can occur anywhere along the path of kidney ascent, from the sacral to the lumbar region.

Abnormal rotation • Abnormal rotation occurs when the kidney fails to rotate or rotates too much during ascent.

Horseshoe kidney • A horseshoe kidney results from fusion of the poles of the kidneys.

Accessory renal arteries • Accessory renal arteries may arise from inadequate regression of caudal vessels during ascent.

Ectopic ureter • An ectopic ureter results in incontinence.

Renal agenesis • Bilateral renal agenesis results in **oligohydramnios** because the fetal kidneys generate amniotic fluid.

Embryonic Sexual Differentiation

• **Gonadal sex** is determined by genes on the sex chromosomes. It refers to the specific path on which undifferentiated gonads embark.
• **Phenotypic sex** is determined by *hormone secretions* of the cells in the gonads.

Primordial Structure	*Female Derivative*	*Male Derivative*
Mesonephric tubules	Epoophoron Paroophoron	Efferent ductules
Wolffian duct (also called the mesonephric duct)	Gartner's duct	Epididymis Vas deferens Seminal vesicles Ejaculation ducts
Müllerian duct (also called the paramesonephric duct)	Fallopian tubes Uterus Upper vagina	Appendix testes
Genital tubercle	Clitoris —Corpus cavernosa —Glans clitoris	Penis —Corpus cavernosa —Glans penis
Urethral folds	Labia minora	Corpus spongiosum
Labioscrotal swellings	Labia majora	Scrotum and ventral epidermis of penis
Urogenital sinus	Paraurethral glands Bartholin's glands Vagina	Prostate gland Cowper's glands Prostatic utricle

Sexual Differentiation

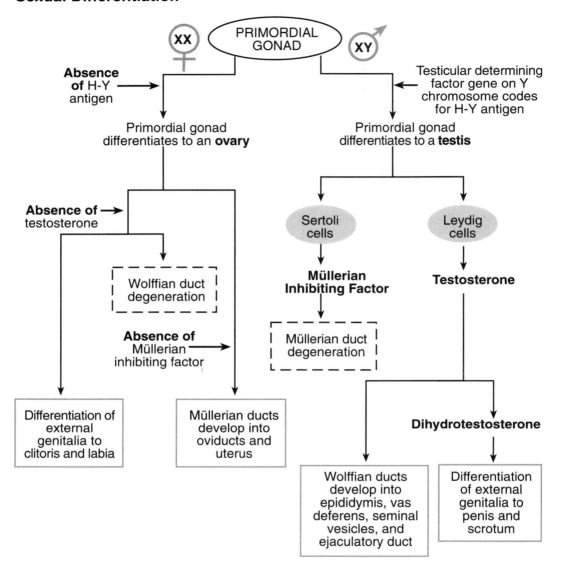

Uterus

- The uterus arises from **paramesonephric ducts** in the absence of **Müllerian inhibiting substance.**

Developmental Defects

Ambiguous genitalia
- Ambiguous genitalia are caused by a defect in the biosynthesis or response to testosterone or dihydrotestosterone. Deficiency of 5-α-reductase or a lack of appropriate receptors will result in partial or complete feminization. Male pseudohermaphrodites results from incomplete masculinization.

Testicular feminization
- Testicular feminization occurs in genetic males deficient in androgen receptors. Patients have normal or elevated androgen levels and complete feminization of external genitalia.

Female pseudohermaphrodism
- Female pseudohermaphrodism occurs in female embryos exposed to androgens. These patients have ovaries, but their genital ducts and external genitalia are either fully or partially male. In adrenogenital syndrome, endogenous androgenic substances from the adrenal cortex cause masculinization. Female pseudohermaphroditism also occurs when exogenous androgenic substances (e.g., progesterone) are given during pregnancy.

True hermaphrodites
- True hermaphrodites possess both ovaries and testes.

Male pseudohermaphrodites
- Male pseudohermaphrodites have testes, but genital ducts and external genitalia are either fully or partially female.

Fetal Brain

- **Hensen's node** is a depression in the primitive streak that gives rise to the notochord and somites.

The Brain Vesicles and their Adult Derivatives

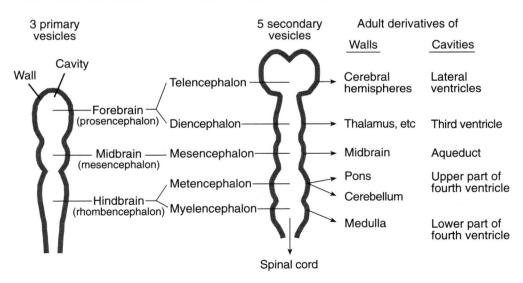

Critical Periods in Gestational Development

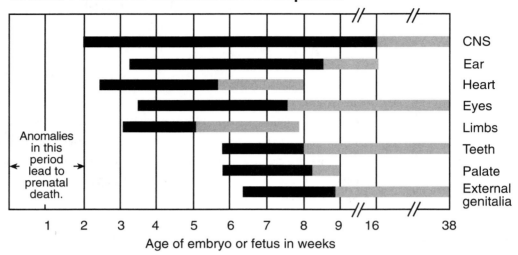

Age of embryo or fetus in weeks

■ Very sensitive periods when teratogens may induce major anamolies
▨ Periods when teratogens may induce minor anamolies

Neural Tube Defects

- Failure of neural folds to fuse dorsally leads to major defects in mesodermal components (meninges, neural arches, epimeric musculature, skin).

- Defects range from complete craniosacral myeloschisis to spina bifida occulta. Meningocele (herniation of meninges through a defect of the skull or spinal cord) and myelomeningocele (herniation of neural tissue as well as meninges) may accompany such defects.

- Anencephaly, caused by failure of neural folds to fuse cranially, is incompatible with life. It is **associated with polyhydramnios.**

- Open defects (e.g., spina bifida) are associated with high maternal α-fetoprotein levels.

Behavioral Science and Epidemiology

<hr>

CHAPTER 9

Coach's Tips

- Behavioral science questions on the USMLE cover a broad range of topics including study design and statistical analysis, epidemiology, human behavior, and basic psychiatric disorders.
- The topic is worth studying. Reviewing behavioral science is quick and high yield.
- Statistics and epidemiology are most important. The definitions of sensitivity, specificity, and so on, come up repeatedly.
- Topics relating to aging are high yield.
- Other high-yield topics include personality disorders, ego defenses, drugs and alcohol, and the sleep cycle.
- A few questions ask for the best way to talk to a given patient. When in doubt, empathize or pick the most open-ended answer.

<hr>

Study Design

Type of Study	Description
Case report	Reports the facts about a single patient
Case series	Reports the facts about a series of patients with a given disease (e.g., 30 patients with paroxysmal nocturnal hemoglobinuria)
Case-control	Reports facts on a group of patients with a condition (e.g., smokers) compared with a group of patients without the condition (e.g., nonsmokers)
Cohort	Reports data on a group followed over time; by definition, a cohort study must report data from at least two distinct points in time • Some review books **erroneously** use the terms "cohort" and "prospective" synonymously. Cohort studies can be **either prospective or retrospective.** • *Mnemonic:* A "cohort" was a unit in the Roman Legion that marched together. Thus, a "cohort study" marches through time.

continued

Type of Study	Description
Cross-sectional	Reports data on a population of people gathered at one point in time; useful for providing descriptions of populations
Experiment	Reports data from a **prospectively** designed experiment with at least one group of patients who underwent an intervention compared with at least one group of patients who were controls
Meta-analysis	**Pools the information from multiple studies** to draw conclusions

- Studies attempt to discern associations (e.g., Is cigarette smoking related to lung cancer?). As in a trial by jury, the purpose of a study is to "convict the guilty" (discover true associations) and "acquit the innocent" (refute false associations).

Statistics

- A **type I error** consists of incorrectly reporting a false finding as true (convicting the innocent). α = percentage chance of making a type I error.
- A **type II error** involves incorrectly reporting a true finding as false (acquitting the guilty). β = percentage chance of making a type II error.
- *Power* describes the ability of a study to detect true findings (i.e., ability of the study to correctly convict the guilty). Power = (1 − β). Studies are usually designed such that power is 80% or greater.

Diagnostic Tests

- The only sure things are death and taxes. Therefore, no test is perfect.

	Has disease	*No disease*
Test positive	a	b
Test negative	c	d

Sensitivity

- Sensitivity is the percentage of people with a disease who test positive for the disease.

sensitivity = a/(a + c)

a = people with disease who test positive

a + c = all people with disease

Specificity • Specificity is the percentage of people without a disease who test negative for the disease (the test indicates they are healthy).

specificity $= d/(b + d)$

d = people without disease who test negative
b + d = all people without disease

Positive Predictive Value • Positive predictive value is the chance that someone who tests positive actually has the disease.

$PPV = a/(a + b)$

a = people with disease who test positive
a + b = all people who test positive

Negative Predictive Value • Negative predictive value is the chance that someone who tests negative is truly healthy.

$NPV = d/(c + d)$

d = people without disease who test negative
c + d = all people who test negative

Reliability Versus Validity • **Reliability** is the reproducibility of a test.
  • *Internal reliability* means that tests results are the same when the test is given by different examiners.
  • *Test-retest reliability* means that similar results are achieved when the same person is tested more than once.
• **Validity** is whether a test assesses what it was designed to assess. Sensitivity and specificity are components of validity.

Risk Factors

	Has disease	No disease
Has risk factor	a	b
No risk factor	c	d

Relative Risk
- **Relative risk** is the chance that someone with a given risk factor has a disease **relative** to the chance of someone without the risk factor.

  RR = [a/(a + b)] / [c/(c + d)]

- Relative risk can be computed only for studies (e.g., cohort or cross-sectional) that have the number of diseased persons in a natural proportion to the number of healthy persons.
- In case-control studies, persons with a disease may be overrepresented in the study group. In such cases, relative risk can be guesstimated by the odds ratio.

  Odds ratio = ad/bc

Tests

- The following tests are used to examine the likelihood that a given result is not due to chance alone. The mathematics involved are very low yield.

T-Tests
- T-tests measure the **difference between two means.**
- A **paired t-test** compares the same group at two points.
- An **independent t-test** compares different groups at one point.

ANOVA Tests
- ANOVA tests are analyses of variance. They compare the differences between the means of more than two groups.

χ^2 (Chi-Squared) Tests
- χ^2 tests the difference between frequencies (percentages) in a sample.

Correlation
- **Correlation** represents the mutual relationship between two continuous variables. The correlation coefficient r has a value between -1 and 1. An r value close to positive or negative 1 indicates a very strong positive or negative correlation, respectively, between two variables. If r = 0, there is no correlation between the variables. Correlation, however strong, **does not imply causality.**

Some Important Definitions

Illusion
- An **illusion** is a misinterpretation of something that is present. *Example:* The patient thinks he sees a panther when a dog walks by.

Hallucination	• **Hallucinations,** on the other hand, are totally invented.
Example:	*The patient sees a panther when there's no dog in sight.*

Delusion	• **Delusions** are blatantly false beliefs.
Example:	*The patient is certain he is a panther and the dog has been sent by the C.I.A. to get him.*

(Beliefs held by large groups of people are not delusions. For example, believing that biochemistry is relevant to medical practice is technically not a delusion.)

Delusions Versus Loose Associations

- Delusions are a disorder of thought *content:* "I am a panther."
- Loose associations are thought shifts that make no sense: "That dog looks like a panther. Do you own a goldfish?"

Personality Disorders

- Personality disorder questions typically describe a patient and ask you to choose a course of action. These can be some of the hardest behavioral medicine questions, but a few clues help.

Dependent

- **Dependent personality** is the favorite. Dependent patients are afraid of being helpless and want to be cared for. The case will likely be a woman who wants the doctor to make decisions for her, who visits the doctor because her spouse told her to, and who needs extra attention when sick.

Approach: *Be reassuring and schedule regular office visits even when the patient is not sick.*

Compulsive

- **Compulsive** patients fear loss of control and may become controlling during illness. They typically experience time urgency. The case will likely be a businessman or other harried professional who demands to make a phone call in the middle of a doctor visit or who wants to know every detail of his disease.

Approach: *Be informative and patient.*

Paranoid

- **Paranoid** patients often blame the doctor for their illnesses. They avoid intimacy and are very sensitive to any perceived lack of attention or caring. The case will likely be a business-like, anxious man who has seen several doctors and who thought that they were all incompetent or insensitive.

Approach: *Be professional, avoid humor, and don't try to be warm.*

Narcissistic
- **Narcissistic** patients often feel their self-image threatened by illness. They tend to overestimate their abilities and cannot tolerate criticism from others. They crave attention and love. The case will likely be a man who demands the best care and who brags.

Approach: *Be careful to avoid implicit criticism.*

Other Personality Disorders
- Other personality disorders require only recognition.
  - Histrionic personalities are colorful and excitable and may make sexual advances toward the doctor or threaten suicide to gain attention. They are usually female.
  - Passive-aggressive personalities often ask for help or advice from the doctor and then don't comply with it.

Defense Mechanisms

- Ego defenses are generally **unconscious** mental efforts to decrease anxiety and maintain self-esteem. Most are self-explanatory and easily remembered. Below are all the frequently tested defenses.

Less Mature Defense Mechanisms

Denial
- Refusing to believe or act on difficult truths (e.g., terminal illness).
  - **Denial is the most common defense mechanism used by patients.**
  - Denial is particularly common in patients with newly diagnosed cancer or AIDS.
  - Noncompliance with medications is a common feature of denial.

Regression
- Responding to stress by acting less mature than usual.
  - **Regression is common in hospitalized patients of all ages.**
  - Young kids may revert to wetting the bed when in the hospital.

Acting out
- Expressing unacceptable feelings in actions.
  - A teenager starts stealing because of conflict at home.

Rationalization
- Using logic to justify actions.

Repression	• **Involuntarily** excluding a feeling from one's consciousness.
Displacement	• Transferring emotions from an unacceptable to an acceptable idea, person, or object.
Dissociation	• Separating the functions of mental processes (e.g., multiple personalities).
Projection	• Attributing unacceptable thoughts or impulses to others.

Mature Defense Mechanisms

Altruism	• Unselfishly assisting those in need.
Humor	• Reducing anxiety by making light of a situation or feeling.
Sublimation	• Channeling unacceptable drives into socially acceptable actions (e.g., exercise or sports).
Suppression	• **Consciously** putting aside unwanted feelings (as opposed to repression, which is unconscious).

Sleep Cycle and Sleep Disorders

• Sleep is divided into five stages that constitute two general categories: REM sleep and non-REM sleep.

Non-REM (Stages 1–4)

• **Decrease** in heart rate, respirations, and blood pressure.
• Episodic body movements occur.
• Stages 3 and 4 of non-REM sleep are **slow** (or **delta**) **wave sleep** and represent the deepest, most relaxed sleep. They are associated with bed wetting (enuresis), somnambulism, and night terrors.

REM

• **Increase** in heart rate, respirations, blood pressure, and brain oxygen consumption.
• The onset of REM sleep normally occurs 90 minutes after falling asleep. REM sleep then occurs at progressively shorter intervals. Most REM sleep occurs in the last third of the night.
• REM sleep is associated with dreaming, penile and clitoral erection, and skeletal muscle paralysis (except for the eye muscles).

Sleep Stage	Wave(s)	EEG Characteristics
Awake	α, β	Beta waves correlate with active mental concentration.
1	α to Θ	Alpha waves disappear and give rise to theta waves (light sleep). Waves are low voltage and high frequency.
2		Sleep spindles, K complexes.
3–4	δ	Slow wave sleep. Delta waves are high voltage (amplitude) and low frequency.
REM	α-like	Low-voltage, high-frequency sawtooth waves that are similar to those seen in the awake state. Dreaming occurs in this stage.

Neurotransmitters Involved in Sleep

- Knowing these makes it easy to remember sleep changes associated with autonomic drugs and disease.

Neurotransmitter	Role in Sleep
Serotonin (5-HT)	Produces sleep
Norepinephrine (NE)	Decreases REM
Acetylcholine (ACh)	Increases REM
Dopamine	Produces wakefulness

Sleep Pattern Changes Associated with Aging and Disease

Factor	Changes
Aging	**Decreased REM and slow wave sleep,** increased sleep latency
Major depression	**Increased REM sleep,** decreased time (increased central ACh) between REM cycles, shift of majority of REM to beginning of the night, decreased REM latency
Alzheimer's disease	**Decreased REM** and slow wave sleep (decreased central ACh)
Narcolepsy	Sleep comes suddenly and REM is entered within a few minutes; may include hypnagogic hallucinations just as one falls asleep

Aging

Life Span • Longevity correlates with parents' life span, **marriage,** and being **female.**

 • Other factors are white race, education, and social support.

 • Women live an average of **8 years longer** than men.

Aging-Related Changes

The physiology of aging is a story of decline.

 • Cardiac output decreases.
 • Basal metabolic rate decreases.
 • Lung volumes (e.g., vital capacity and functional reserve capacity) decrease.
 • Memory, calculation ability, and response time decrease.
 • Learning is impaired.
 • Muscle bulk and strength decrease.
 • Sexual function declines, although interest often remains.
 • In women, vaginal tone, lubrication, and barrel length decrease.
 • In men, ejaculation and erection take longer and are less intense.
 • **Intelligence remains approximately the same** (unless mental illness occurs).

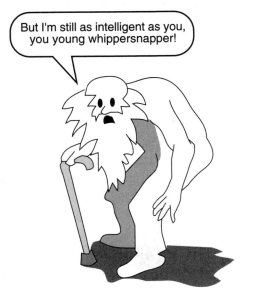

Mental disease
increases with age
- **Depression** is common.
- **Suicide** is twice as common in the elderly.
- **Alzheimer's disease is the most important cause of dementia.**
  - Generalized cerebral atrophy occurs.
  - Neurofibrillary **tangles** and neuritic **plaques** are seen in brain stains.
  - Abnormal amyloid may play a major role.
  - Fewer neurons are found in the nucleus basalis of Meynert.

Physical disease
increases with age
- Heart disease, cancer, and stroke all increase with age.

Issues Concerning the Aging

- The Eriksonian task for the elderly is ego integrity versus despair.
- Elisabeth Kübler-Ross described the process of dying (and grieving) in five stages.
  - Bargaining, denial, anger, acceptance, and depression can occur in any order or simultaneously.

Mnemonic: *In other words, "You **B**e **DAAD**" ("be dead").*

- **Medicare** provides hospital and medical costs for all persons **over 65** and persons of any age with debilitating illness or **permanent disability.**

Epidemiology

Schizophrenia
- Lifetime prevalence of 1.5%
- Genetic influence
- Occurs equally in blacks and whites, men and women

Infant Mortality Rate
- Average in U.S. (1990) is 9.2 per 1000.
- Rate among blacks is twice the rate among whites.
- Rate among Native Americans is 14 per 1000.

Intelligence Quotient (IQ)
- IQ is 100 × (mental age/chronologic age). If mental age is equal to chronologic age, IQ is 100 (average).
- Standard deviation (SD) is 10; 3 SDs below the mean (IQ $\leq 2\ 70$) indicates mental retardation.
- IQ remains stable through adulthood.
- Intelligence tests are influenced by cultural biases.

Epidemiology of Death

- The top three killers in the United States are:

  1) **Heart disease**
  2) Cancer
  3) Stroke

- Cancer deaths are further broken down by gender.

Rank	Men	Women
1	Lung cancer	Lung cancer
2	**Prostate cancer**	**Breast cancer**
3	Colon cancer	Colon cancer

- **Injuries** are the leading cause of death in people aged 1 to 24.

Mnemonic: **A**dolescents die in **A**ccidents.

- Injuries are also the leading cause of death in 25- to 44-year old men, as of October 1997. Previous to this, in the earlier 1990s, AIDS was the leading killer.
- The top killer of infants is congenital anomalies.

Miscellaneous

- **Advance directives are binding.** Do what they say.
- Good Samaritan laws apply to **M.D.s** and in some states to other health care professionals. These laws provide some protection against malpractice suits in emergency situations.
- Confidentiality is breachable in cases of **child abuse, threat to life** (of patient or other person), certain communicable diseases such as HIV, and emergencies.
- To commit a patient for involuntary treatment, the patient must be mentally ill *and* either a danger to self or others or unable to obtain food and shelter.
- Drug dependence (e.g., to benzodiazepines) is best predicted by a history of alcoholism.

Pathology

CHAPTER 10

Todd C. Brady

_____ **Coach's Tips**

- Several pathology questions will give a clinical history and ask for the most likely diagnosis. The patient's age, sex, race, and presentation will all be classic for the disease.
- Pathology questions commonly come with pictures. Read the text first. The pictures are often redundant.
- The #1 cause of cancer for various ages and organs is high yield.
- Risk factors for common diseases such as arteriosclerosis, hypertension, lung cancer, breast cancer, colon cancer, stroke, and diabetes are high yield.
- If a single lab test can virtually diagnose a disease, it is high yield. An example is d-dimers for disseminated intravascular coagulation.
- Pathology due to altered physiology is high yield.

Mechanisms of Cell Injury

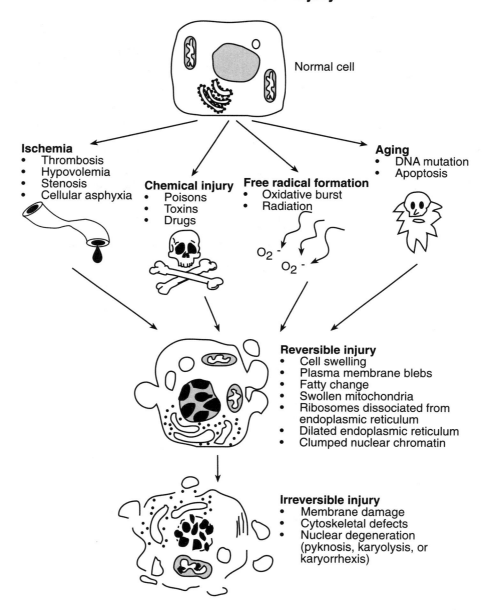

Normal cell

Ischemia
- Thrombosis
- Hypovolemia
- Stenosis
- Cellular asphyxia

Chemical injury
- Poisons
- Toxins
- Drugs

Free radical formation
- Oxidative burst
- Radiation

O_2^-

O_2^-

Aging
- DNA mutation
- Apoptosis

Reversible injury
- Cell swelling
- Plasma membrane blebs
- Fatty change
- Swollen mitochondria
- Ribosomes dissociated from endoplasmic reticulum
- Dilated endoplasmic reticulum
- Clumped nuclear chromatin

Irreversible injury
- Membrane damage
- Cytoskeletal defects
- Nuclear degeneration (pyknosis, karyolysis, or karyorrhexis)

Cell Death

Types of Necrosis

Coagulative
- Associated with ischemic cell death as it occurs in myocardial infarction; basic cell structures are initially preserved.

Liquefactive
- Found in brain infarcts or bacterial abscesses; cell structures are obliterated.

Caseous
- Results from *Mycobacterium tuberculosis* infection (white, cheesy).

Fat, enzymatic
- Results from intrapancreatic or intraperitoneal release of digestive enzymes.

Fibrinoid
- Associated with thrombosis and inflammation as in vasculitis.

Hemorrhagic
- Results from disruption of vascular integrity and subsequent infarction of the affected tissue.

Apoptosis (Programmed Cell Death)
- Chromatin condenses.
- Cytoplasmic blebs form.
- DNA fragmentation ("laddering") occurs.

Inflammation

Inflammatory Mediators

Mediator	Class	Function
IL-1, TNF-α < IFN-γ	Cytokines	Chemotaxis and activation of leukocytes
C5a	Complement	Chemotaxis, vasodilation
Histamine, serotonin	Vasoactive amines	Vasodilation, increase in permeability
Nitric oxide	Free radical	Vasodilation
Bradykinin	Kinin	Vasodilation, increase in vessel permeability
Thromboxane (TXA$_2$)	Arachidonic acid metabolite	Vasoconstriction
Prostacyclin (PGI$_2$)	Arachidonic acid metabolite	Vasodilation
Leukotrienes	Arachidonic acid metabolite	Vasoconstriction, chemotaxis

Inflammation

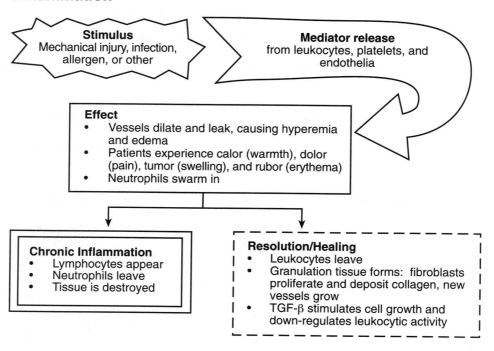

Stimulus
Mechanical injury, infection, allergen, or other

Mediator release
from leukocytes, platelets, and endothelia

Effect
- Vessels dilate and leak, causing hyperemia and edema
- Patients experience calor (warmth), dolor (pain), tumor (swelling), and rubor (erythema)
- Neutrophils swarm in

Chronic Inflammation
- Lymphocytes appear
- Neutrophils leave
- Tissue is destroyed

Resolution/Healing
- Leukocytes leave
- Granulation tissue forms: fibroblasts proliferate and deposit collagen, new vessels grow
- TGF-β stimulates cell growth and down-regulates leukocytic activity

Infection

Suppurative Inflammation

- Suppurative inflammation is initially marked by neutrophil aggregation and accumulation. Abscesses may result as bacterially infected tissue is destroyed by the release of proteases and oxidative metabolites. Gram-positive and gram-negative bacteria can cause suppurative inflammation.

Lymphocytic Infiltration

- Suggests a viral infection.

Granulomatous Inflammation

- Granulomatous inflammation is marked by mononuclear phagocytes. The agents tend to be intracellular organisms (e.g., mycobacteria and spirochetes). Multinucleate giant cells may be found.

Granulomatous Reactions

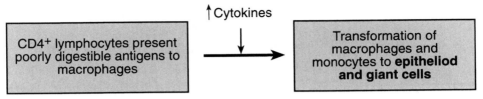

CD4$^+$ lymphocytes present poorly digestible antigens to macrophages

↑Cytokines

Transformation of macrophages and monocytes to **epitheliod and giant cells**

Metabolic Acidosis Secondary to Shock

How Does Shock Lead to Metabolic Acidosis?

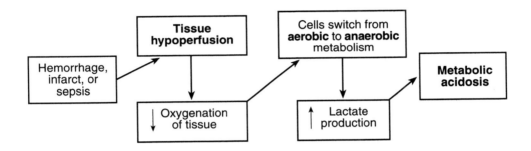

Hemorrhage, infarct, or sepsis

Tissue hypoperfusion

↓ Oxygenation of tissue

Cells switch from **aerobic** to **anaerobic** metabolism

↑ Lactate production

Metabolic acidosis

Defects in Host Defense

- **Chediak-Higashi Syndrome** is an autosomal recessive disease of defective microtubule polymerization. Poor phagocytosis results from impaired fusion of phagosomes with lysosomes.
- **Complement deficiency**
  - C5a deficiency results in a chemotaxis defect.
  - C5-8 deficiency results in an inability to form the membrane attack complex, making patients susceptible to *Neisseria* infections.
- **Chronic granulomatous disease**
  - Deficiency in NADPH oxidase prevents formation of the super-oxide needed to kill bacteria, causing susceptibility to bacterial infection.
- **Myeloperoxidase deficiency**
  - Defect in the enzyme that produces hypochlorite leads to impaired ability to kill certain bacterial and *Candida* species.

Hypersensitivity

- **Type I (anaphylactic)** is due to binding of antigen to pre-formed antibody bound to the surface of mast cells and basophils. It is marked by vasodilation and increased vascular permeability.
- **Type II (antibody-mediated)** is due to pre-formed antibody in the blood. It results in lysis or phagocytosis of antibody-coated cells.
- **Type III (immune complex formation)** comes in two forms:
  1) **Serum sickness** is a systemic disease caused by the formation of circulating immune complexes that deposit into tissues (e.g., kidneys, joints, and small vessels).
  2) **Local immune complex disease (Arthus reaction)** is similar to serum sickness except it is localized to a specific area. Severe necrotizing vasculitis can occur with fibrinoid necrosis and accumulation of neutrophils.
- **Type IV (T-cell mediated)** has two important features:
  1) **Delayed type hypersensitivity** is mediated by CD4-positive T-cells and has an 8- to 12-hour delay from the onset of exposure to antigen.
  2) Cytotoxicity is mediated by CD8-positive T cells that kill antigen-bearing target cells.
- The PPD skin test for tuberculosis exposure is a classic example of type IV hypersensitivity.

Transplant Rejection

- Transplant rejection is divided into four types:
  1) **Hyperacute rejection** occurs within minutes in individuals who have pre-formed antibody against the foreign antigen.
  2) **Accelerated acute rejection** occurs days to months after transplantation secondary to the development of antibodies against the transplanted organ.
  3) **Acute rejection** occurs months after transplantation and is T cell mediated. It responds to immunosuppressive therapy.
  4) **Chronic rejection** is a progressive tissue rejection that does not respond to immunosuppression. The cause is not well established.
- **Graft-versus-host disease** is a special form of rejection in which donor T cells react against the immune-deficient host.

Erythroblastosis Fetalis

- Erythroblastosis fetalis is hemolytic anemia due to blood group incompatibility between a mother and a fetus. Rh-negative mothers of

Rh-positive fetuses should receive anti-D globulin (Rhogam) immediately after delivery to prevent erythroblastosis fetalis in the subsequent fetus. Affected fetuses show enlargement of the liver and spleen and severe hyperbilirubinemia.

Autoimmune Diseases

- **Grave's disease** is caused by autoantibodies that activate the thyroid-stimulating hormone receptor leading to hyperthyroidism. It occurs most commonly in middle-aged women and often presents with exophthalmos.
- **Hashimoto's thyroiditis** is caused by autoantibodies against microsomal components. It is the most common cause of hypothyroidism. Patients have enlarged thyroid glands and may have been previously thyrotoxic. Thyroid tissues show extensive infiltration of lymphocytes, plasma cells, and macrophages.
- **Myasthenia gravis** is caused by autoantibodies against acetylcholine receptors in the neuromuscular end plate. Classically, women during the third decade of life present with thymic enlargement and use-dependent muscle weakness.
- **Eaton-Lambert syndrome** produces symptoms similar to myasthenia gravis, but the autoantibodies are directed against proteins involved in intracellular calcium release.
- **Systemic lupus erythematosus** (SLE) is a common disease, affecting 1 in 2500. **Females are affected ten times as often as males,** and blacks are affected more often than whites. Onset is usually in the second or third decade of life. **Autoantibodies against double-stranded DNA** and ribonucleoprotein (Smith) antigens are most common. Symptoms include a butterfly rash, photosensitivity, oral ulcers, pericarditis, mental illness, and renal disease. Drugs (e.g., **procainamide** and **hydralazine**) can trigger a lupus syndrome.
- **Systemic sclerosis (scleroderma)** causes diffuse inflammation and fibrosis throughout the body. Hypergammaglobulinemia, antinuclear antibodies, and rheumatoid factor are commonly present. Some patients get the CREST syndrome (**c**alcinosis, **R**aynaud's phenomenon, **e**sophageal dysmotility, **s**clerodactyly, and **t**elangiectasia).
- **Goodpasture's syndrome** is caused by autoantibodies against the basement membrane of the kidneys and lungs.
- **Dermatomyositis** presents with rash around the eyes and knuckles. Patients have bilateral proximal muscle weakness from shoulders down to the distal extremities. **Polymyositis** is similar to dermatomyositis but without the skin findings.

- **Sjögren's syndrome** is also known as sicca syndrome because it causes dry eyes and mouth. Inflammation of the lacrimal and salivary glands occurs and antinuclear and antiribonucleoprotein antibodies (Ro and La) appear.
- **Rheumatoid arthritis (RA)** is a systemic inflammatory disease characterized by non-suppurative inflammation of the joints and other tissues. **Rheumatoid factor** (autoantibodies against the Fc portion of IgG) appears in the synovial fluid of most affected patients. Onset is highest in women 20 to 40 years of age. RA is characterized by chronic synovitis with the formation of granulation tissue (pannus). Inflammation destroys articular cartilage and causes ulnar deviation of the fingers. Rheumatoid nodules afflict up to 50% of patients with rheumatoid arthritis. The etiology remains unclear.

Immune Deficiencies

- **DiGeorge's syndrome** results from defects in the development of the third and fourth pharyngeal pouches. The thymus and parathyroids fail to develop, leading to tetany (due to hypocalcemia from absence of parathyroid hormone) and absence of cell-mediated immunity.
- **Bruton's X-linked agammaglobulinemia** is characterized by absence of circulating B cells and very low serum IgG. Patients experience recurrent bacterial infections with encapsulated bacteria.
- **Wiskott-Aldrich syndrome** is an X-linked recessive disease marked by the triad of eczema, thrombocytopenia, and recurrent infections by encapsulated bacteria as well as fungi, viruses, and protozoa. Cell-mediated immunity is impaired and T-cell counts eventually diminish.
- **Severe combined immunodeficiency (SCID)** is characterized by defective T- and B-cell functions. Patients may lack both T and B cells and die within 1 year of birth. Half of these patients lack adenosine deaminase.
- **IgA deficiency** is the most common immunodeficiency, but most individuals are asymptomatic.

Neoplasia

- **Neoplasia** means "new growth." Neoplasms are unresponsive to normal growth control regulation, and exhibit numerous abnormal characteristics:
  - **Decreased growth factor requirements**
  - **Loss of contact inhibition** (normal cell growth slows when cells touch)

- **Anchorage independence** (normal cells often require extracellular matrix foundations for growth)
- **Altered expression of extracellular matrix** (e.g., fibronectin) and cell-cell or cell-matrix binding proteins (e.g., Cadherins, integrins)
- **Decreased cell division time**
- **Disorganized microfilament bundles** (e.g., actin stress fibers)
- **Increased secretion of proteases** (e.g., plasminogen activator)
- **Increased secretion of angiogenic growth factors** (e.g., vascular endothelial growth factor and fibroblast growth factor)

Morphology
- **Metaplasia** is a change in cell type from one to another (e.g., squamous to columnar).
- **Dysplasia** describes cells that have a variety of shapes and sizes and that are not in their usual orientation in the tissue. Tissues that are dysplastic do not necessarily progress to become neoplastic.
- **Anaplasia** is a lack of consistent differentiation of cells (wide variety of sizes, shapes, and stages of cell cycle). It is the defining characteristic of malignant neoplasms.
- **Metastasis** is a second distinct site of cancer that originated from the primary site. A tumor that has metastasized is unequivocally malignant. **Lymphogenous** metastases are found in lymph nodes throughout the body. **Hematogenous** metastases are commonly found in the liver, lungs, and brain.

The Most Common Malignant Cancers

Organ	Cancer (listed from most frequent to least frequent)
Lung	Squamous cell carcinoma > Adenocarcinoma > Small cell Carcinoma
Colon	Adenocarcinoma
Prostate	Adenocarcinoma
Breast	Infiltrating ductal carcinoma > Infiltrating lobular carcinoma
Cervix	Squamous cell carcinoma
Pancreas	Adenocarcinoma
Urinary tract	Transitional cell carcinoma > Renal cell carcinoma
Ovary	Epithelial (e.g., serous) > Germ cell (e.g., Teratoma)
Testicle	Germ cell (e.g., embryonal) > Interstitial cell (e.g., Leydig)
Uterus	Adenocarcinoma

continued

Organ	Cancer (listed from most frequent to least frequent)
Brain	Astrocytoma > Metastatic > Meningioma
Esophagus	Squamous cell carcinoma > > Adenocarcinoma
Liver	Metastasis > > Hepatocellular carcinoma
Thyroid	Papillary carcinoma > Follicular carcinoma (both are rare)
Bone	Metastasis > > Osteosarcoma > Chondrosarcoma > Ewing's tumor
Skin	Basal cell carcinoma > Squamous cell carcinoma > Melanoma

Paraneoplastic Syndromes

Syndrome	Cause	Cancer
Cushingoid	ACTH-like substance	Lung small cell carcinoma
Neural Disorders	Probably immunologic	Lung small cell, thymoma
Carcinoid	Vasoactive amines, kinins	Bronchial, pancreatic cancer
Hypercalcemia	PTH-like substance	Lung squamous carcinoma
Venous thrombosis	Hypercoagulable state	Pancreatic carcinoma

Tumor Markers

Marker	Tumors
CEA	Carcinoma of the colon and other gastrointestinal malignancies
PSA	Prostate adenocarcinoma
α-Fetoprotein	Hepatocellular carcinoma, yolk sac tumor, malignant teratoma
β-hCG	Choriocarcinoma
α_1-antitrypsin	Liver and yolk sac tumors
CA-125	Ovarian cancer
S-100	Melanoma, neural tumors

Vascular Pathology

Edema

- Localized **edema** is due to an imbalance of fluids entering and exiting tissue (e.g., hypertension, congestive heart failure, hyperaldosteronism, nephrotic syndrome, deep vein thrombosis, lymphedema).

- **Anasarca** is generalized edema. **Ascites** is free fluid within the peritoneal cavity.

Embolism

- A **dislodged thrombus** is the most common type of embolism. Venous emboli from deep veins of the legs commonly lodge in the pulmonary tree (pulmonary embolism). Factors predisposing to venous thrombi include stasis (e.g., sitting immobile for a long period of time on a plane or lying immobile in bed when sick), vessel endothelial injury, and a hypercoagulable state (e.g., oral contraceptives or paraneoplastic syndrome).

- **Air emboli (Caisson disease)** occur most commonly in deep-sea divers.
- **Fat emboli** occur 1 to 3 days after fractures of long bones.
- **Amniotic fluid emboli** occur as the result of prolonged labor and are commonly associated with disseminated intravascular coagulation.
- **Paradoxical embolus** is a venous thrombus that enters the arterial tree as a result of right-to-left shunt in the heart (e.g., a patent foramen ovale).

Pathologic Changes During Myocardial Infarction

Time After Infarct	Gross Pathology	Microscopic Pathology
0 to 0.5 hour	None	Reversible injury: mitochondrial swelling, slight fiber distortion
1 to 2 hours	None	Irreversible injury: disruption of sarcolemma
4 to 12 hours	None	Edema, hemorrhage, condensation of chromatin
24 to 72 hours	Pallor	Coagulation necrosis, neutrophil influx
10 days	Center of infarct is soft, reddish-yellow or brown, sometimes with hyperemic border	Necrotic cellular resorption by macrophages; fibrovascular regeneration leading to scarring

Other Diseases of Coagulation

- Clot formation is a balance between procoagulants and anticoagulants.
- **Budd-Chiari syndrome** is thrombosis of the major hepatic veins.
- **Disseminated intravascular coagulopathy** (DIC) is a consumption coagulopathy commonly caused by sepsis or toxin ingestion. Because coagulation compounds are rapidly used up in the formation of microthrombi, a **hypo**coagulable state eventually results. **D-dimers are elevated.**
- **Immune thrombocytopenic purpura** is an autoimmune disease involving antiplatelet antibodies.

Coagulation Defects

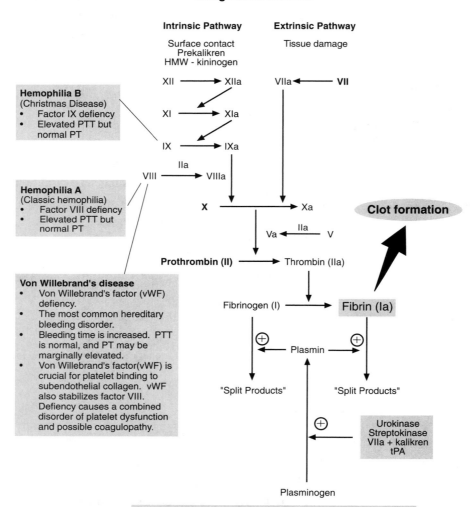

Hemophilia B
(Christmas Disease)
- Factor IX defiency
- Elevated PTT but normal PT

Hemophilia A
(Classic hemophilia)
- Factor VIII defiency
- Elevated PTT but normal PT

Von Willebrand's disease
- Von Willebrand's factor (vWF) defiency.
- The most common hereditary bleeding disorder.
- Bleeding time is increased. PTT is normal, and PT may be marginally elevated.
- Von Willebrand's factor(vWF) is crucial for platelet binding to subendothelial collagen. vWF also stabilizes factor VIII. Defiency causes a combined disorder of platelet dysfunction and possible coagulopathy.

Intrinsic Pathway

Surface contact
Prekalikren
HMW - kininogen

XII ⟶ XIIa

XI ⟶ XIa

IX ⟶ IXa

VIII ⟶ VIIIa
(IIa)

X ⟶ Xa

Extrinsic Pathway

Tissue damage

VIIa ⟵ **VII**

Clot formation

Va ⟵ V
(IIa)

Prothrombin (II) ⟶ Thrombin (IIa)

Fibrinogen (I) ⟶ **Fibrin (Ia)**

⊕ ⟵ Plasmin ⟶ ⊕

"Split Products"   "Split Products"

⊕ ⟵ Urokinase
Streptokinase
VIIa + kalikren
tPA

Plasminogen

Prothrombin (II), VII, XI, X: Depend on **vitamin K** for activation; their synthesis is inhibited by **coumadin**.

Genetic Diseases

Diseases of Aneuploidy

Aneuploidy involves having a number of chromosomes that is not a multiple of the normal haploid number n. For humans, $n = 23$.

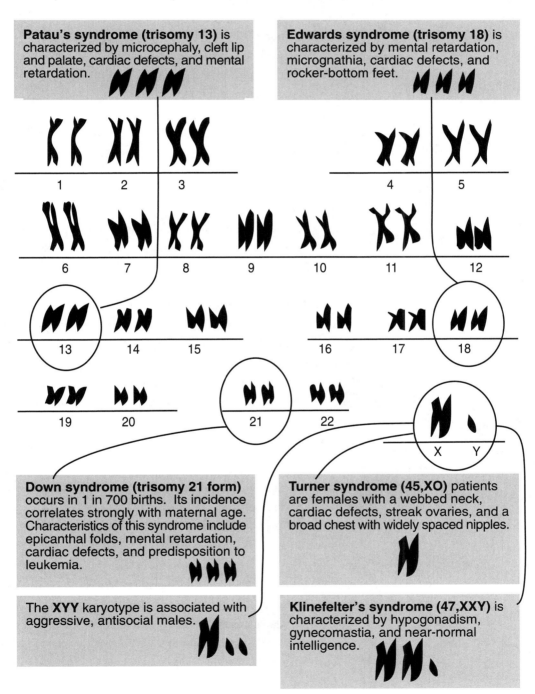

Patau's syndrome (trisomy 13) is characterized by microcephaly, cleft lip and palate, cardiac defects, and mental retardation.

Edwards syndrome (trisomy 18) is characterized by mental retardation, micrognathia, cardiac defects, and rocker-bottom feet.

Down syndrome (trisomy 21 form) occurs in 1 in 700 births. Its incidence correlates strongly with maternal age. Characteristics of this syndrome include epicanthal folds, mental retardation, cardiac defects, and predisposition to leukemia.

Turner syndrome (45,XO) patients are females with a webbed neck, cardiac defects, streak ovaries, and a broad chest with widely spaced nipples.

The **XYY** karyotype is associated with aggressive, antisocial males.

Klinefelter's syndrome (47,XXY) is characterized by hypogonadism, gynecomastia, and near-normal intelligence.

Autosomal Dominant

- **Familial hypercholesterolemia** occurs in 1 in 500 persons. An absent or defective LDL receptor predisposes to early atherosclerosis.
- **Huntington's disease** leads to late-onset choreiform movements and dementia. The caudate and putamen are affected. The responsible defect is on chromosome 4.
- **Adult polycystic kidney disease** is a chromosome 16 defect. Berry aneurysms occur in 10% to 30% of patients.
- **Marfan's syndrome** is believed to be a defect in fibrillin. Dissecting aortic aneurysms, floppy cardiac valves, tall stature, and subluxation of the lens occur.
- **Neurofibromatosis**
  - **Type 1 (von Recklinghausen's disease)** is characterized by multiple neurofibromas, pigmented skin (café-au-lait spots), and Lisch nodules.
  - **Type 2** is characterized by bilateral acoustic neuromas.
- **Retinoblastoma** results from a defective cancer suppressor gene. Patients have an increased risk for osteosarcoma and breast carcinoma. **Knudsen's two-hit hypothesis** proposes that since every individual has two copies of the genes for Rb, both copies must be knocked out for the cell to lose Rb function and become malignant. As a result of a **germline mutation,** individuals may inherit one copy of the defective gene. The remaining normal copy then undergoes **somatic mutation** (mutation after fertilization), leading to **loss of heterozygosity** and malignancy.
- **Ehlers-Danlos syndromes** encompass many disease subtypes involving defects in collagen synthesis and structure. Findings include "stretchy" skin, loose joints, and spontaneous rupture of arteries. Lysyl oxidase deficiency is one etiology.

Autosomal Recessive

- **Adenosine deaminase deficiency** causes 50% of autosomal recessive severe combined immunodeficiency. T-cell function is impaired, impairing B-cell function as well.
- **Tay-Sachs disease** occurs frequently in Ashkenazi Jews (1 in 30 are carriers). A β-hexosaminidase A deficiency leads to excess GM2 gangliosides in the CNS, causing mental retardation and early death.
- **Phenylketonuria (PKU)** is due to phenylalanine hydroxylase deficiency. Untreated patients develop mental retardation and a musty odor. Mothers with PKU should reduce dietary phenylalanine when pregnant. Dietary restriction of phenylalanine is also the treatment of choice for infants.

- **Galactosemia** results from deficiency in either galactose-1-phosphate uridyl transferase or galactokinase. Hepatomegaly, cataracts, and mental retardation are observed. Infants experience failure to thrive, diarrhea, jaundice, and vomiting. Treatment involves dietary restriction of galactose.
- **Cystic fibrosis** is most common in Caucasians. **Defective chloride ion transport** leads to recurrent pulmonary infection, pancreatic insufficiency, and diabetes. An increased sweat chloride is diagnostic. Mothers of children with cystic fibrosis often report that their babies taste salty.

X-Linked
- **Duchenne muscular dystrophy** is a defect in the gene encoding dystrophin, a cytoskeletal protein. Patients experience progressive muscle weakness, pseudohypertrophy of calf muscles, and eventually respiratory difficulty with death by age 20.
- **Lesch-Nyhan syndrome** is a defect in hypoxanthine guanine phosphoribosyl transferase (HGPRT) affecting the purine salvage pathway. Excess uric acid secretion, self-mutilation, and mental retardation are observed with HGPRT deficiency.
- **Glucose-6-phosphate dehydrogenase deficiency** causes hemolytic anemia due to reduced ability of red cells to protect themselves from oxidative injury. Antimalarials and sulfonamides can trigger hemolysis.

Enzyme Deficiencies
- α_1-**Antitrypsin deficiency** results in pulmonary emphysema, liver injury, and increased risk for hepatocellular cancer.
- **21-Hydroxylase deficiency** is the most common steroid enzyme defect. Patients have defects in cortisol and mineralocorticoid synthesis and have an elevated ACTH level.
- **Tyrosinase** deficiency leads to albinism.

Environmental

Carcinogens
- **Smoking** causes emphysema and chronic bronchitis and increases the risk for atherosclerosis, bronchogenic carcinoma, and cancer of the oral cavity, esophagus, pancreas, and bladder. The urine test for smoking is for nicotine, but the main urine carcinogen is nitrosamines. On stopping smoking, the risk for heart disease decreases to about normal in a matter of weeks to years, and the risk for lung cancer decreases to about normal after approximately 10 years.

- **Asbestos** increases the risk for bronchogenic carcinoma (especially in smokers) and **mesothelioma.** Asbestosis is characterized by dyspnea, cough, and interstitial pulmonary fibrosis associated with ferruginous bodies (rod-like fibers that contain iron). Shipyard and construction workers are at risk for asbestos exposure.
- **Oral contraceptives** (synthetic estradiol and/or progestin) increase the risk of cervical cancer and venous thrombosis, especially in conjunction with smoking.
- **Aflatoxin** is produced by Aspergillus species. It increases the risk for hepatocellular carcinoma.
- **Aromatic amines** increase the incidence of transitional cell bladder carcinoma in workers exposed to aniline dye and rubber manufacturing.
- **Ultraviolet radiation** damages DNA by forming pyrimidine dimers. UV light dramatically increases the risk of skin cancer in patients with xeroderma pigmentosum (a defect in the DNA excision repair system). UV exposure increases the risk of squamous cell and basal cell carcinomas as well as melanoma.

Poisons
- **Carbon tetrachloride** in small doses causes fatty change in the liver. In large doses it causes CNS depression and liver destruction.
- **Carbon monoxide** avidly displaces oxygen from hemoglobin.
- **Alcohol** causes liver cirrhosis, GI bleeding, Wernicke-Korsakoff syndrome (nystagmus, ataxia, dementia), cardiomyopathy, pancreatitis, and fetal alcohol syndrome.
- **Mercuric chloride** binds to cell membranes causing increased membrane permeability and inhibition of ATPase-dependent transport.
- **Lead** binds disulfide groups to inactivate proteins. Especially damaging to the developing CNS, lead exposure leads to demyelination and decreased IQ as well as multiorgan damage, anemia, and "lead lines" on gums.

Nutrition

Vitamin Deficiencies

Vitamin	*Effects of Deficiency*
A (retinol)	Dry eyes, night blindness, immune defects
B_1 (thiamine)	Beri-beri ("wet": cardiomyopathy, "dry": poly neuropathy), Wernicke-Korsakoff syndrome
B_3 (niacin)	Pellagra and the three Ds (**dementia, dermatitis, diarrhea**)

continued

Vitamin	Effects of Deficiency
B$_6$ (pyridoxine)	Glossitis, peripheral neuropathy, dermatitis
B$_{12}$ (cyanocobalamin)*	Macrocytic, megaloblastic anemia with motor and postural nerve deficits. Hypersegmented neutrophils are diagnostic of B$_{12}$ deficiency. This syndrome is called **pernicious anemia** when production of **intrinsic factor,** which allows B$_{12}$ to be absorbed, is insufficient or defective.
C (ascorbic acid)	Scurvy is due to defective collagen synthesis. Patients have poor wound healing, swollen gums, and bruises.
D	Children get rickets and adults get osteomalacia.
E	Degeneration of axons in the posterior columns of the spinal cord
K	Bleeding is due to the inability to synthesize clotting factors II, VII, IX, and X and proteins C and S.

*In contrast, folic acid (folate) deficiency results in a macrocytic, megaloblastic anemia without neurologic deficit.

Protein Deficiencies

- **Kwashiorkor's syndrome** occurs when there is a greater deficiency in proteins than calories. Dependent edema and liver enlargement are the results.
- **Marasmus** is a calorie deficiency defined as being less than 60% of the normal weight for the patient's age and height.

Trace Metal Deficiencies

- **Iron** deficiency is the leading cause of microcytic anemia in infants and the elderly.
- **Zinc** deficiency leads to growth retardation and infertility.
- **Iodine** deficiency causes goiter and hypothyroidism.

Aging-Related Processes

- **Calcification** occurs around cardiac valves, in arterial walls, and at sites of previous injuries (e.g., pancreatitis, atherosclerosis, and pulmonary fibrosis).
- Lean and total body **weight decreases** with age while the proportion of body fat increases.
- **Osteoporosis** occurs most severely in postmenopausal women. Estrogen replacement therapy and calcium supplements slow the progression of osteoporosis.

Idiopathic Processes

- **Amyloidosis** is the deposition of amyloid proteins in multiple organ systems, most commonly in the heart, spleen, liver, and kidney. Associated diseases include multiple myeloma and senility. Amyloid proteins stained with Congo red exhibit green birefringence under polarized light.

- **Sarcoidosis** is characterized by multiple noncaseating granulomas in various organ systems. It is more common in African Americans. Patients can present with lymphadenopathy, hepatomegaly, splenomegaly, cough, or any of a wide variety of symptoms.

Bodies, Inclusions, and Funny Cells

Disease	Pathologic Finding
DIC	D-dimers and fibrin split products
Rheumatic heart disease	Aschoff bodies (granulomas with giant cells) and Anichkov (Anitschkow) cells (histiocytes around the granulomas)
Multiple myeloma	Russell bodies (Ig inclusions within plasma cells)
Alcoholic hepatitis	Mallory bodies (hyaline)
Parkinson's disease	Lewy bodies (intracytoplasmic, eosinophilic bodies)
Hodgkin's disease	Reed-Sternberg cells (owl-eye cells)
Wilson's disease	Mallory bodies (eosinophilic bodies surrounding the nucleus) in the liver
SLE	Wire loop lesions in the kidney
AML	Auer rods in granulocytes or myeloblasts
Rabies virus	Negri bodies (eosinophilic)
Chlamydia	Glycogen-containing inclusions
Cytomegalovirus	Intranuclear inclusions
Atherosclerosis	Foam cells (lipid-laden macrophages)
Sarcoid	Multinucleate giant cells with cytoplasmic asteroid bodies
Papilloma virus	Koilocytosis (perinuclear vacuolization)
G6PD deficiency	Heinz bodies (precipitated hemoglobin in erythrocytes)

Similar Disease Comparisons

- Many diseases are similar to one another. The differences between these diseases appear often on the Boards.

Type I Diabetes

- Onset usually during childhood
- Pancreas eventually ceases insulin production inappropriate amounts
- Insulin therapy required
- Predisposes to ketoacidosis

Type II Diabetes

Onset usually during adulthood

Pancreas releases insulin, but at inappropriate times and in

Insulin may or may not be required

Associated with obesity

Hodgkin's Lymphoma

- Associated with the Reed-Sternberg Cell
- Responds well to radiation therapy
- Median age in the 30s
- Usually confined to lymphoid tissues

Non-Hodgkin's Lymphoma

Multiple forms

Responds best to chemotherapy, but prognosis can be poor

Median age in the 60s, but younger onset in AIDS patients

Solid organ metastasis

Acute Leukemia

- Composed of immature lymphocytic precursors (leukemic blasts)
- *Lymphoblastic form:* affects children median age > 50
- *Myeloblastic form:* affects middle-aged adults

Chronic Leukemia

Composed of relatively mature leukocytic precursors

Lymphocytic form: B cell origin

Myeloid form: granulocytic stem cell median age = 40–50

Lung Small Cell Carcinoma

- Interstitial Carcinoma of lymphocyte-like cells ("oat cells")
- Metastasizes rapidly and widely, involving mediastinal and hilar lymph nodes
- Prominent neuroendocrine paraneoplastic syndromes

Lung Squamous Cell Carcinoma

Bronchogenic Carcinoma associated with "keratin pearls"

Metastasizes slowly outside the thorax, well-localized tumors

Fewer paraneoplastic manifestations

continued

Crohn's Disease
- Alternating normal and affected areas of bowel ("skip lesions")
- Small intestine and colon often affected

Ulcerative Colitis

Starts in the rectum and ascends without skip lesions

The colon is exclusively affected.

Crohn's Disease
- Transmural fibrosis, fissuring necrosis
- Causes fistulae (skin, bladder)

Ulcerative Colitis

Only the mucosa and sub-mucosa are affected

Flattened mucosa with pseudopolyps

Restrictive Lung Disease
- Soft tissue or musculo-skeletal defect resulting in decreased lung compliance
- Decreased total lung volume

- Normal or high FEV1/FVC ratio
- Interstitial thickening (between capillaries and airspace), decreased diffusion
- Caused by ARDS, sarcoid, scoliosis

Obstructive Lung Disease

Reduction of airflow, usually on expiration, through bronchial tree

Increased total lung volume, increased expiration time

Low FEV1/FVC ratio

Possible smooth muscle hyper-trophy, interstitial inflamma-tion, alveolar destruction

Caused by asthma, emphysema, cystic fibrosis

Nephrotic Syndrome
- Proteinuria
- Hypoalbuminemia
- Generalized edema
- Hyperlipidemia and lipiduria

Nephritic Syndrome

Hematuria

Oliguria

Azotemia

Hypertension

Skin Squamous Cell Carcinoma
- Arise from epidermal squames
- Begins as red-brown plaque that enlarges to form a rimmed necrotic ulcer
- Metastasis follows penetration of dermal basement membrane

Skin Basal Cell Carcinoma

Arise from basal cells around pilosebaceous glands

Begins as pale papule that slowly progresses to form an ulcer

Metastasis almost never occurs

Review Books: Student Evaluations

Due to the inordinate number of review books on the market for the USMLE Step 1, it is often difficult for students to decide on which review books to use for the Boards. A further complication is that different persons tend to like different books.

As a means to help the student choose books, we conducted a student survey to evaluate the top-selling review books on the market. We surveyed over 180 students from more than 50 different medical schools who had prepared for the USMLE Step 1. To our knowledge, none of the student volunteers were affiliated with any publishing companies nor were they otherwise contributors to Crashing the Boards.

Methods and Explanations

- The surveys asked the students to evaluate the books on a five point scale as follows:
  1. Not useful, not relevant, or has too many drawbacks.
  2. Has some uses, but also some major problems.
  3. A solid, useful book.
  4. A really good book. Well worth using.
  5. A great book! Can't go wrong!

- Students separately evaluated the usefulness of the book as a Boards review book (**Rating for the Boards**) or as a textbook (**Rating as a Textbook**). For each book and category, we calculate the mean rating (**Avg. Score**) and plot the corresponding histogram based on all valid responses. The total number of responses in each case are listed in the column titled "*n*" for number.

- In addition, we compiled all of the written comments from surveyed students and present them as **Candid Student Comments.** These comments are unedited and uncensored except in the rare case where they would be defaming and not publishable.

- *Write-ins:* Many students wrote in and evaluated books they liked but that were not in the original survey. These books were therefore appended to the compiled list and are marked by the words "*Write-in*" in the margin notes. Obviously, for these books, there are fewer responses than for other books.

- *Coach's hints:* In a few instances, we write in comments to clear up points of confusion. We distinguish these comments from the **Candid Student Comments** by prefacing them with the *"Coach's hint"* marker.

General Pointers
- A common mistake is to bite off more than you can chew. Choose books and materials that you can comfortably read and master.
- Before you purchase a book, take a moment to browse the book and see if it suits you. The choice of books and resources ultimately depends on your own goals and personality.

General Review Books

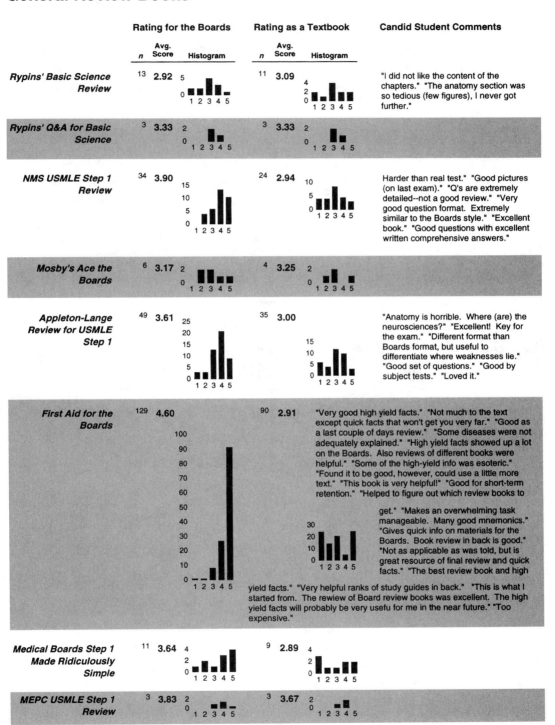

	Rating for the Boards			Rating as a Textbook			Candid Student Comments
	n	Avg. Score	Histogram	n	Avg. Score	Histogram	
Rypins' Basic Science Review	13	2.92		11	3.09		"I did not like the content of the chapters." "The anatomy section was so tedious (few figures), I never got further."
Rypins' Q&A for Basic Science	3	3.33		3	3.33		
NMS USMLE Step 1 Review	34	3.90		24	2.94		Harder than real test." "Good pictures (on last exam)." "Q's are extremely detailed--not a good review." "Very good question format. Extremely similar to the Boards style." "Excellent book." "Good questions with excellent written comprehensive answers."
Mosby's Ace the Boards	6	3.17		4	3.25		
Appleton-Lange Review for USMLE Step 1	49	3.61		35	3.00		"Anatomy is horrible. Where (are) the neurosciences?" "Excellent! Key for the exam." "Different format than Boards format, but useful to differentiate where weaknesses lie." "Good set of questions." "Good by subject tests." "Loved it."
First Aid for the Boards	129	4.60		90	2.91		"Very good high yield facts." "Not much to the text except quick facts that won't get you very far." "Good as a last couple of days review." "Some diseases were not adequately explained." "High yield facts showed up a lot on the Boards. Also reviews of different books were helpful." "Some of the high-yield info was esoteric." "Found it to be good, however, could use a little more text." "This book is very helpful!" "Good for short-term retention." "Helped to figure out which review books to get." "Makes an overwhelming task manageable. Many good mnemonics." "Gives quick info on materials for the Boards. Book review in back is good." "Not as applicable as was told, but is great resource of final review and quick facts." "The best review book and high yield facts." "Very helpful ranks of study guides in back." "This is what I started from. The rewiew of Board review books was excellent. The high yield facts will probably be very usefu for me in the near future." "Too expensive."
Medical Boards Step 1 Made Ridiculously Simple	11	3.64		9	2.89		
MEPC USMLE Step 1 Review	3	3.83		3	3.67		

Anatomy

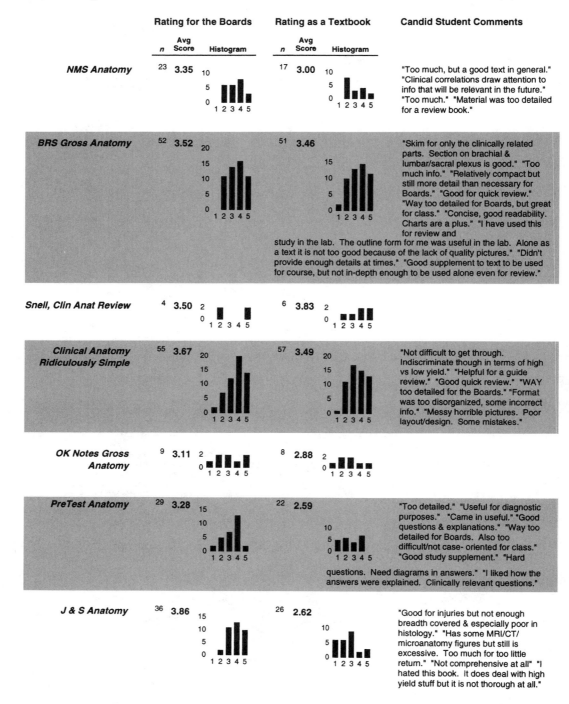

	Rating for the Boards			**Rating as a Textbook**			**Candid Student Comments**
	n	Avg Score	Histogram	*n*	Avg Score	Histogram	
NMS Anatomy	23	3.35		17	3.00		"Too much, but a good text in general." "Clinical correlations draw attention to info that will be relevant in the future." "Too much." "Material was too detailed for a review book."
BRS Gross Anatomy	52	3.52		51	3.46		"Skim for only the clinically related parts. Section on brachial & lumbar/sacral plexus is good." "Too much info." "Relatively compact but still more detail than necessary for Boards." "Good for quick review." "Way too detailed for Boards, but great for class." "Concise, good readability. Charts are a plus." "I have used this for review and study in the lab. The outline form for me was useful in the lab. Alone as a text it is not too good because of the lack of quality pictures." "Didn't provide enough details at times." "Good supplement to text to be used for course, but not in-depth enough to be used alone even for review."
Snell, Clin Anat Review	4	3.50		6	3.83		
Clinical Anatomy Ridiculously Simple	55	3.67		57	3.49		"Not difficult to get through. Indiscriminate though in terms of high vs low yield." "Helpful for a guide review." "Good quick review." "WAY too detailed for the Boards." "Format was too disorganized, some incorrect info." "Messy horrible pictures. Poor layout/design. Some mistakes."
OK Notes Gross Anatomy	9	3.11		8	2.88		
PreTest Anatomy	29	3.28		22	2.59		"Too detailed." "Useful for diagnostic purposes." "Came in useful." "Good questions & explanations." "Way too detailed for Boards. Also too difficult/not case-oriented for class." "Good study supplement." "Hard questions. Need diagrams in answers." "I liked how the answers were explained. Clinically relevant questions."
J & S Anatomy	36	3.86		26	2.62		"Good for injuries but not enough breadth covered & especially poor in histology." "Has some MRI/CT/ microanatomy figures but still is excessive. Too much for too little return." "Not comprehensive at all" "I hated this book. It does deal with high yield stuff but it is not thorough at all."

Biochemistry

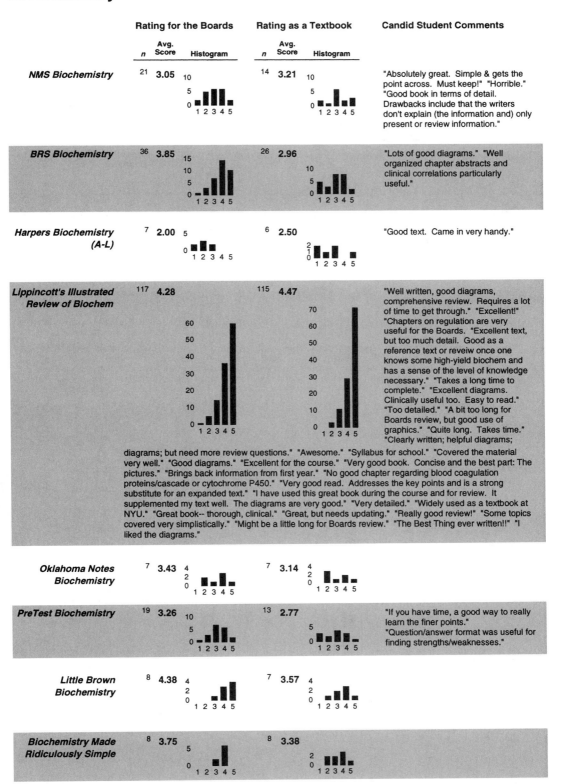

	Rating for the Boards			Rating as a Textbook			Candid Student Comments
	n	Avg. Score	Histogram	n	Avg. Score	Histogram	
NMS Biochemistry	21	3.05		14	3.21		"Absolutely great. Simple & gets the point across. Must keep!" "Horrible." "Good book in terms of detail. Drawbacks include that the writers don't explain (the information and) only present or review information."
BRS Biochemistry	36	3.85		26	2.96		"Lots of good diagrams." "Well organized chapter abstracts and clinical correlations particularly useful."
Harpers Biochemistry (A-L)	7	2.00		6	2.50		"Good text. Came in very handy."
Lippincott's Illustrated Review of Biochem	117	4.28		115	4.47		"Well written, good diagrams, comprehensive review. Requires a lot of time to get through." "Excellent!" "Chapters on regulation are very useful for the Boards. "Excellent text, but too much detail. Good as a reference text or reveiw once one knows some high-yield biochem and has a sense of the level of knowledge necessary." "Takes a long time to complete." "Excellent diagrams. Clinically useful too. Easy to read." "Too detailed." "A bit too long for Boards review, but good use of graphics." "Quite long. Takes time." "Clearly written; helpful diagrams;

diagrams; but need more review questions." "Awesome." "Syllabus for school." "Covered the material very well." "Good diagrams." "Excellent for the course." "Very good book. Concise and the best part: The pictures." "Brings back information from first year." "No good chapter regarding blood coagulation proteins/cascade or cytochrome P450." "Very good read. Addresses the key points and is a strong substitute for an expanded text." "I have used this great book during the course and for review. It supplemented my text well. The diagrams are very good." "Very detailed." "Widely used as a textbook at NYU." "Great book-- thorough, clinical." "Great, but needs updating." "Really good review!" "Some topics covered very simplistically." "Might be a little long for Boards review." "The Best Thing ever written!!" "I liked the diagrams."

	Rating for the Boards			Rating as a Textbook			Candid Student Comments
Oklahoma Notes Biochemistry	7	3.43		7	3.14		
PreTest Biochemistry	19	3.26		13	2.77		"If you have time, a good way to really learn the finer points." "Question/answer format was useful for finding strengths/weaknesses."
Little Brown Biochemistry	8	4.38		7	3.57		
Biochemistry Made Ridiculously Simple	8	3.75		8	3.38		

Behavioral Science

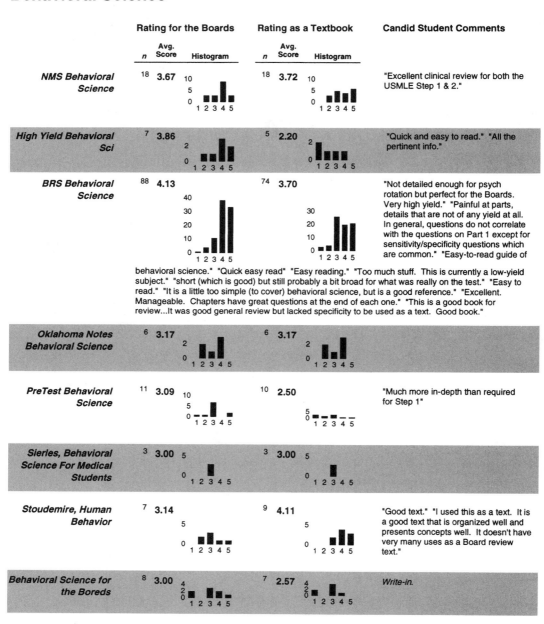

	Rating for the Boards			Rating as a Textbook			Candid Student Comments
	n	Avg. Score	Histogram	n	Avg. Score	Histogram	
NMS Behavioral Science	18	3.67		18	3.72		"Excellent clinical review for both the USMLE Step 1 & 2."
High Yield Behavioral Sci	7	3.86		5	2.20		"Quick and easy to read." "All the pertinent info."
BRS Behavioral Science	88	4.13		74	3.70		"Not detailed enough for psych rotation but perfect for the Boards. Very high yield." "Painful at parts, details that are not of any yield at all. In general, questions do not correlate with the questions on Part 1 except for sensitivity/specificity questions which are common." "Easy-to-read guide of

behavioral science." "Quick easy read" "Easy reading." "Too much stuff. This is currently a low-yield subject." "short (which is good) but still probably a bit broad for what was really on the test." "Easy to read." "It is a little too simple (to cover) behavioral science, but is a good reference." "Excellent. Manageable. Chapters have great questions at the end of each one." "This is a good book for review...It was good general review but lacked specificity to be used as a text. Good book."

Oklahoma Notes Behavioral Science	6	3.17		6	3.17		
PreTest Behavioral Science	11	3.09		10	2.50		"Much more in-depth than required for Step 1"
Sierles, Behavioral Science For Medical Students	3	3.00		3	3.00		
Stoudemire, Human Behavior	7	3.14		9	4.11		"Good text." "I used this as a text. It is a good text that is organized well and presents concepts well. It doesn't have very many uses as a Board review text."
Behavioral Science for the Boreds	8	3.00		7	2.57		Write-in.

Microbiology

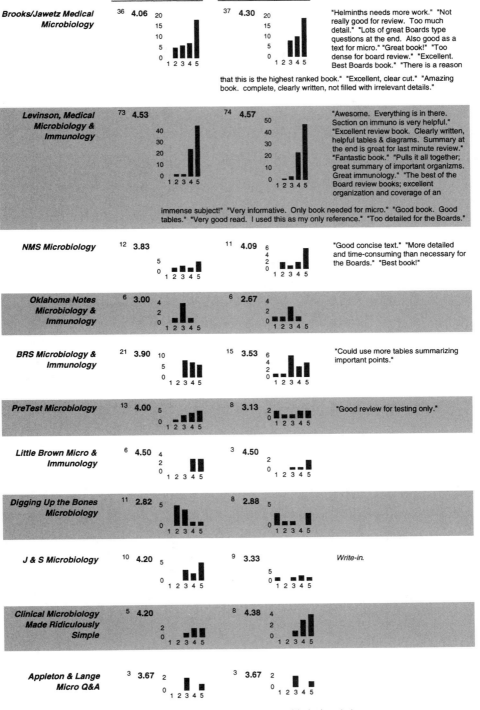

	Rating for the Boards			Rating as a Textbook			Candid Student Comments
	n	Avg. Score	Histogram	n	Avg. Score	Histogram	

Brooks/Jawetz Medical Microbiology — Rating for the Boards: n 36, 4.06; Rating as a Textbook: n 37, 4.30

"Helminths needs more work." "Not really good for review. Too much detail." "Lots of great Boards type questions at the end. Also good as a text for micro." "Great book!" "Too dense for board review." "Excellent. Best Boards book." "There is a reason that this is the highest ranked book." "Excellent, clear cut." "Amazing book. complete, clearly written, not filled with irrelevant details."

Levinson, Medical Microbiology & Immunology — Rating for the Boards: n 73, 4.53; Rating as a Textbook: n 74, 4.57

"Awesome. Everything is in there. Section on immuno is very helpful." "Excellent review book. Clearly written, helpful tables & diagrams. Summary at the end is great for last minute review." "Fantastic book." "Pulls it all together; great summary of important organizms. Great immunology." "The best of the Board review books; excellent organization and coverage of an immense subject!" "Very informative. Only book needed for micro." "Good book. Good tables." "Very good read. I used this as my only reference." "Too detailed for the Boards."

NMS Microbiology — Rating for the Boards: n 12, 3.83; Rating as a Textbook: n 11, 4.09

"Good concise text." "More detailed and time-consuming than necessary for the Boards." "Best book!"

Oklahoma Notes Microbiology & Immunology — Rating for the Boards: n 6, 3.00; Rating as a Textbook: n 6, 2.67

BRS Microbiology & Immunology — Rating for the Boards: n 21, 3.90; Rating as a Textbook: n 15, 3.53

"Could use more tables summarizing important points."

PreTest Microbiology — Rating for the Boards: n 13, 4.00; Rating as a Textbook: n 8, 3.13

"Good review for testing only."

Little Brown Micro & Immunology — Rating for the Boards: n 6, 4.50; Rating as a Textbook: n 3, 4.50

Digging Up the Bones Microbiology — Rating for the Boards: n 11, 2.82; Rating as a Textbook: n 8, 2.88

J & S Microbiology — Rating for the Boards: n 10, 4.20; Rating as a Textbook: n 9, 3.33

Write-in.

Clinical Microbiology Made Ridiculously Simple — Rating for the Boards: n 5, 4.20; Rating as a Textbook: n 8, 4.38

Appleton & Lange Micro Q&A — Rating for the Boards: n 3, 3.67; Rating as a Textbook: n 3, 3.67

Coach's hint. Many students confuse the Jawetz and the Levinson texts because both are blue and Jawetz co-authored the Levinson text. We suggest using the Levinson text rather than Jawetz for Boards purposes.

Pathology

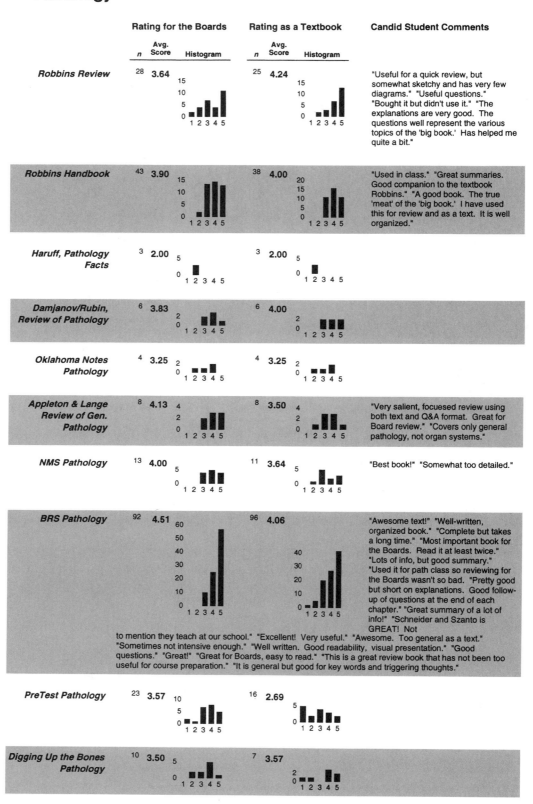

	Rating for the Boards			**Rating as a Textbook**			**Candid Student Comments**
	n	Avg. Score	Histogram	n	Avg. Score	Histogram	
Robbins Review	28	3.64		25	4.24		"Useful for a quick review, but somewhat sketchy and has very few diagrams." "Useful questions." "Bought it but didn't use it." "The explanations are very good. The questions well represent the various topics of the 'big book.' Has helped me quite a bit."
Robbins Handbook	43	3.90		38	4.00		"Used in class." "Great summaries. Good companion to the textbook Robbins." "A good book. The true 'meat' of the 'big book.' I have used this for review and as a text. It is well organized."
Haruff, Pathology Facts	3	2.00		3	2.00		
Damjanov/Rubin, Review of Pathology	6	3.83		6	4.00		
Oklahoma Notes Pathology	4	3.25		4	3.25		
Appleton & Lange Review of Gen. Pathology	8	4.13		8	3.50		"Very salient, focuesed review using both text and Q&A format. Great for Board review." "Covers only general pathology, not organ systems."
NMS Pathology	13	4.00		11	3.64		"Best book!" "Somewhat too detailed."
BRS Pathology	92	4.51		96	4.06		"Awesome text!" "Well-written, organized book." "Complete but takes a long time." "Most important book for the Boards. Read it at least twice." "Lots of info, but good summary." "Used it for path class so reviewing for the Boards wasn't so bad. "Pretty good but short on explanations. Good follow-up of questions at the end of each chapter." "Great summary of a lot of info!" "Schneider and Szanto is GREAT! Not
PreTest Pathology	23	3.57		16	2.69		
Digging Up the Bones Pathology	10	3.50		7	3.57		

to mention they teach at our school." "Excellent! Very useful." "Awesome. Too general as a text." "Sometimes not intensive enough." "Well written. Good readability, visual presentation." "Good questions." "Great!" "Great for Boards, easy to read." "This is a great review book that has not been too useful for course preparation." "It is general but good for key words and triggering thoughts."

Pharmacology

	Rating for the Boards			Rating as a Textbook			Candid Student Comments
	n	Avg. Score	Histogram	*n*	Avg. Score	Histogram	

Lippincott's Illustrated Review of Pharmacology
n 92 Avg. Score 4.28
n 92 Avg. Score 4.29

"Clear discussions of mechanisms, indications, side effects, etc. of drugs." "Covers maybe too many drugs in each class but very useful drugs and charts." "Very clear and easy to understand. I wish I had used it as a text during pharm instead of waiting for the Boards. Need to start early--this book takes a while to read." "I found this extremely useful." "Great for overview for the Boards. Too simple for the rigors of a course." "I used this during pharm." ""Excellent. I used it for my text for class and for review." "All I needed for my pharm class." "Excellent course review." "Good book. It covers the topics well. Great format and very readable content and time-wise." "Very detailed."

Katzung Basic & Clinical Pharmacology
n 56 Avg. Score 3.94
n 54 Avg. Score 4.06

"Good explanations & the questions were like the Board." "Only use as a reference." "Takes a long time, very detailed." "Occasionally too detailed for Boards. "Way too much to study for Boards unless one is to take several months." "Very concise. Good overview." "Good in conjunction with textbook. Helpful charts." "Also a great book. Readable chapters and good charts." "This is a great book that I use consistently to study for pharm. It is very good." "Supplements the Appleton & Lange book very well."

NMS Pharmacology
n 7 Avg. Score 3.71
n 8 Avg. Score 4.38

Oklahoma Notes Pharmacology
n 5 Avg. Score 4.00
n 4 Avg. Score 3.75

"Good review book. Geared toward Board relevant material. Compact. Focused."

BRS Pharmacology
n 16 Avg. Score 4.00
n 9 Avg. Score 3.56

"Too few tables."

Pharmcards
n 20 Avg. Score 3.75
n 22 Avg. Score 3.64

PreTest Pharmacology
n 20 Avg. Score 3.15
n 17 Avg. Score 2.82

Digging Up the Bones Pharmacology
n 9 Avg. Score 2.89
n 7 Avg. Score 2.43

Clinical Pharmacology Made Ridiculously Simple
n 18 Avg. Score 3.83
n 18 Avg. Score 3.56

"Needs revision." "Oversimplified, so had some erroneous information."

Physiology

	Rating for the Boards			Rating as a Textbook			Candid Student Comments
	n	Avg. Score	Histogram	n	Avg. Score	Histogram	
Ganong Review of Medical Physiology	29	3.41		29	4.14		"Wonderful text but too textbook-like for review." "Too dense for Boards review." "Terrible. Too detailed." "Very helpful for my clinical science and my neuroscience course."
Oklahoma Notes Physiology	4	3.25		4	3.75		
NMS Physiology	29	3.72		28	3.89		"Not too good. Way too many mathematical equations for the Boards & very difficult to read." "Some good chapters but overall not good." "Large and detailed, but useful as a reference. Good drawings/diagrams." "Fairly complete, clear review. Somewhat time-consuming but probably worth it for Boards." "Great text! May be too long and organization is complex--otherwise '5'." " My favorite review book." "Complete. Dense. Needs more questions though." "Better text than review book because there was too much information." "Too much for the Boards." "Used for GI physiology. Good but too long, too few topics."
Little Brown Physiology	2	4.50		3	4.00		"Too many errors, not current enough." "Too wordy for Board review and questions not in appropriate format."
PreTest Physiology	21	4.00		18	3.53		"Good overview questions for basic physiology, but not enough information to use as a text."
BRS Physiology	58	4.33		53	3.80		"Excellent." "Excellent." "Good diagrams. Covers the basics of physiology." "very good. Quick and painless." "Brief, good for succinct review, but at times lacking sufficient detail." "Good." "Easy reading." "Good book. Could use more diagrams. High yield." "Good, to the point." "Can learn important info quickly." "Not enough detail." "Great book--nice review."
Clinical Physiology Made Ridiculously Simple	4	3.50		7	3.79		

Histology/Cell Biology

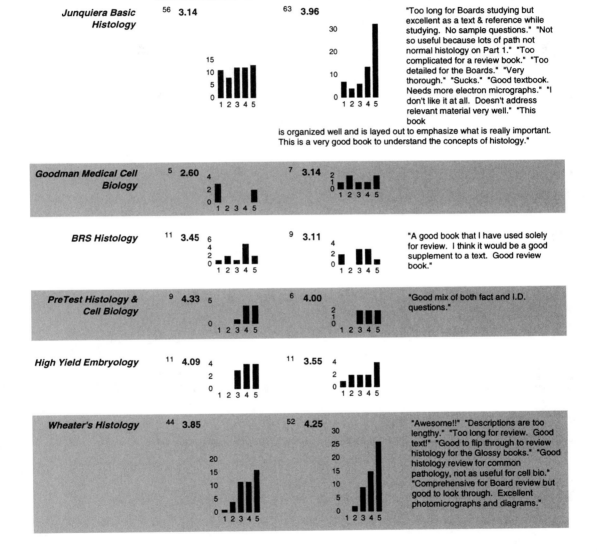

Rating for the Boards — n, Avg. Score, Histogram

Rating as a Textbook — n, Avg. Score, Histogram

Candid Student Comments

Junquiera Basic Histology
n 56, Avg. Score 3.14
n 63, Avg. Score 3.96

"Too long for Boards studying but excellent as a text & reference while studying. No sample questions." "Not so useful because lots of path not normal histology on Part 1." "Too complicated for a review book." "Too detailed for the Boards." "Very thorough." "Sucks." "Good textbook. Needs more electron micrographs." "I don't like it at all. Doesn't address relevant material very well." "This book is organized well and is layed out to emphasize what is really important. This is a very good book to understand the concepts of histology."

Goodman Medical Cell Biology
n 5, Avg. Score 2.60
n 7, Avg. Score 3.14

BRS Histology
n 11, Avg. Score 3.45
n 9, Avg. Score 3.11

"A good book that I have used solely for review. I think it would be a good supplement to a text. Good review book."

PreTest Histology & Cell Biology
n 9, Avg. Score 4.33
n 6, Avg. Score 4.00

"Good mix of both fact and I.D. questions."

High Yield Embryology
n 11, Avg. Score 4.09
n 11, Avg. Score 3.55

Wheater's Histology
n 44, Avg. Score 3.85
n 52, Avg. Score 4.25

"Awesome!!" "Descriptions are too lengthy." "Too long for review. Good text!" "Good to flip through to review histology for the Glossy books." "Good histology review for common pathology, not as useful for cell bio." "Comprehensive for Board review but good to look through. Excellent photomicrographs and diagrams."

Neuroanatomy

	Rating for the Boards			Rating as a Textbook			Candid Student Comments
	n	Avg. Score	Histogram	n	Avg. Score	Histogram	
NMS Neuroanatomy	5	3.40		6	3.50		
BRS Neuroanatomy	16	3.63		19	3.79		"O.K." "This is a good review book -- very complete. Outline form is very useful."
DeGroot Correlative Neuroanatomy	5	3.20		6	3.67		
Barr The Human Nervous System	4	4.25		6	4.33		
PreTest Neuroscience	10	3.60		7	3.00		"Difficult but good."
Clinical Neuroanatomy Made Ridiculously Simple	70	4.23		68	4.10		"Quite useful. Has all the basics." "Helpful for covering main tracts in the nervous system. Some useful mnemonics." "High yield." "Some areas are confusing but overall succinct and helpful." "Reviewed some critical things, e.g. areas of brain supplied by various arteries and circle of willis." "Great basic review of neuro but not overly specific to Boards Q's, especially since no cell bio." "I LOVE

this book--you can read it in a day and learn so much from it." "Good review and concise." "Great conceptual review however more clinical than useful for Step 1. Deficient in anatomic details." "Easy to understand." "Great." "Great book but too detailed for Boards." "Great diagrams." "Excellent approach to a very difficult subject. Good summaries. Makes concepts easy to understand." "Messy drawings."

Oklahoma Notes Neuroanatomy	3	3.67		3	3.67		
High-Yield Neuroanatomy	21	4.48		17	4.03		"Nice high-yield format."

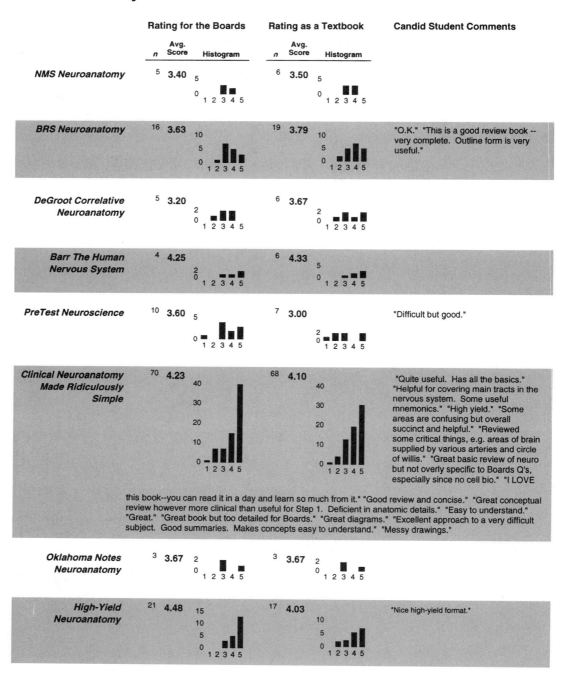

Index

Page numbers set in *italics* denote figures

About the Editors

Principal editor Ben Yeh (guard, Harvard College) earned a reputation on the court as a defensive sparkplug and served a similar role in this project as its guiding influence. After completing his medicine internship at Beth Israel Hospital, he went to UCSF to pursue the family business of radiology. Residency lottery pick Sean Wu (guard, Stanford), master of ball control and student organization, recently completed his grueling PhD work in the Duke Department of Pathology and will continue on at Duke as a resident in internal medicine. Ketan "Shoot for Three" Bulsara (center, Davidson) and Shankha Biswas (forward, North Carolina) proved to be a potent combination in the paint and in the drafts for several sections of this book. Ketan and Shankha are fellow residents at Duke in neurosurgery and cardiothoracic surgery, respectively. Matt Flynn (forward, Harvard), who wore several hats for this work, completed his internship in medicine at UCSF and is now in dermatology residency at Stanford. Lawrence Liao (guard and coach, Duke) completed his internal medicine residency at Vanderbilt. Now he boomerangs back to Duke as a cardiology fellow. Back-up point man Joe Paydarfar (guard, Duke) consistently energized this project much as he did when inserted to run our offense. He is currently a resident in otolaryngology at Washington University.